The Invisible Work of Nurses

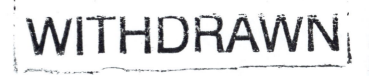

Nursing is typically understood, and understands itself, as a care-giving occupation. It is through its relationships with patients – whether these are absent, present, good, bad or indifferent – that modern day nursing is defined. Yet nursing work extends far beyond direct patient care activities. Across the spectrum of locales in which they are employed, nurses, in numerous ways, support and sustain the delivery and organisation of health services. In recent history, however, this wider work has generally been regarded as at best an adjunct to the core nursing function, and at worse responsible for taking nurses away from their 'real work' with patients. Beyond its identity as the 'other' to care-giving, little is known about this element of nursing practice.

Drawing on extensive observational research of the everyday work in a UK hospital, and insights from practice-based approaches and actor network theory, the aim of this book is to lay the empirical and theoretical foundations for a reappraisal of the nursing contribution to society by shining a light on this invisible aspect of the nursing role. Nurses, it is argued, can be understood as focal actors in health systems who, through myriad processes of 'translational mobilisation', sustain the networks through which care is organised. Not only is this work an essential driver of action, it also operates as a powerful countervailing force to the centrifugal tendencies inherent in healthcare organisations which, for all their gloss of order and rationality, are in reality very loose arrangements.

The Invisible Work of Nurses will be of interest to academics and students across a number of fields, including nursing, medical sociology, organisational studies, health management, science and technology studies and improvement science.

Davina Allen is Professor of Health Service Delivery at Cardiff University, UK. She is Deputy Editor-in-Chief of *Sociology of Health and Illness*.

LIVERPOOL JMU LIBRARY

3 1111 01502 0728

Routledge Advances in Health and Social Policy

New titles

Health Care Reform and Globalisation
The US, China and Europe in comparative perspective
Edited by Peggy Watson

Power and Welfare
Understanding citizens' encounters with state welfare
Nanna Mik-Meyer and Kaspar Villadsen

International Perspectives on Elder Abuse
Amanda Phelan

Mental Health Services for Vulnerable Children and Young People
Supporting children who are, or have been, in foster care
Michael Tarren-Sweeney and Arlene Vetere

Providing Compassionate Health Care
Challenges in policy and practice
Edited by Sue Shea, Robin Wynyard and Christos Lionis

Teen Pregnancy and Parenting
Rethinking the myths and misperceptions
Keri Weed, Jody S. Nicholson and Jaelyn R. Farris

The Invisible Work of Nurses
Hospitals, organisation and healthcare
Davina Allen

Domestic Violence in Diverse Contexts
A re-examination of gender
Sarah Wendt and Lana Zannettino

WITHDRAWN

Professor Davina Allen invites our attention to the real 'organising' work of nurses. She writes to help us 'see', knowing that seeing involves more than the work of an eye. It involves preparing ourselves to notice, recognise, interpret the 'reality' we engage. She invites the reader's preparation for 'seeing' the heretofore invisible nurse work by sharing insight into the relationships and activities that comprise the 'organising work' of front-line hospital nurses – in the simple, complicated and complex systems of modern hospitals.

She clearly explains the theories that underlie what she has noticed and is trying to understand. She describes the care she took in her observations and interpretations. The way she names what she sees and illustrates her points with data from her observational study invites the reader's curiosity about the phenomena.

She weaves her knowledge of the nurse's work and her knowledge of the sociologist's theories and methods together to create a tapestry that attracts the serious student of health care change and improvement today. It deserves the attention of health care leaders and improvers everywhere.

The future redesign of health care requires an understanding of the 'real' work, so that new approaches can be more than hopes and dreams. Allen's observations and interpretations form an important contribution to the development of that understanding.

Paul Batalden, MD
Professor Emeritus, The Dartmouth Institute,
Geisel School of Medicine at Dartmouth College, USA
Senior Fellow, Institute for Healthcare Improvement

The eyes see only what the mind is prepared to comprehend.
Henri Bergson

The Invisible Work of Nurses

Hospitals, organisation
and healthcare

Davina Allen

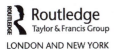
Routledge
Taylor & Francis Group

LONDON AND NEW YORK

First published 2015
by Routledge
2 Park Square, Milton Park, Abingdon, Oxfordshire OX14 4RN

and by Routledge
711 Third Avenue, New York, NY 10017

First issued in paperback 2016

Routledge is an imprint of the Taylor & Francis Group, an informa business

© 2015 Davina Allen

The right of Davina Allen to be identified as author of this work has been asserted by her in accordance with sections 77 and 78 of the Copyright, Designs and Patents Act 1988.

All rights reserved. No part of this book may be reprinted or reproduced or utilised in any form or by any electronic, mechanical, or other means, now known or hereafter invented, including photocopying and recording, or in any information storage or retrieval system, without permission in writing from the publishers.

Trademark notice: Product or corporate names may be trademarks or registered trademarks, and are used only for identification and explanation without intent to infringe.

British Library Cataloguing in Publication Data
A catalogue record for this book is available from the British Library

Library of Congress Cataloging in Publication Data
Allen, Davina, 1963- author.
The invisible work of nurses : hospitals, organisation and healthcare / Davina Allen.
p. ; cm. -- (Routledge advances in health and social policy)
Includes bibliographical references.
I. Title. II. Series: Routledge advances in health and social policy.
[DNLM: 1. Nursing Staff, Hospital--Great Britain. 2. Nursing Process--Great Britain. 3. Nursing Theory--Great Britain. WY 125]
RT89
362.17′3--dc23
2014011167

ISBN 13: 978-1-138-21361-6 (pbk)
ISBN 13: 978-0-415-72325-1 (hbk)

Typeset in Sabon
by Saxon Graphics Ltd, Derby

Contents

Fieldnote conventions

[…] words, phrases or sentences omitted
((material added by the author to make the context/meaning clear))
'words used by study participants'
Data have been edited to preserve anonymity
All names of people and places are pseudonyms

Foreword

This is an important book. It is rare that a book comes along, which reframes the way we look at our world but this is a ground-breaking volume. By using the word 'look' though we are already revealing how powerful and pervasive visual metaphors are as a heuristic device to describe not only what meets the eye but what goes beyond to create meaning. Nurses often complain their work is invisible and of the difficulty of describing what they do. Davina Allen has done us a great service by providing us with a lens through which to 'see' nurses' organising work. This is no mean feat, one which is rigorously grounded in an empirical reconceptualisation of nursing work and draws deftly on actor network theory. Nursing is relational and not just of people. The role that nurses play is often connecting different parts of the system that have or need to have some relationship with each other. This is more than coordination, joining the dots of services making them whole and coherent, but aligning services to patients across time amd space in order to make the system possible in an environment that is complex and in constant churn. As John Berger, the art critic reminds us, 'ways of seeing' are the product of habit and convention. This book stretches our canvass beyond the familiar essentialist conceptions of nursing by bringing the organising work of nurses to the foreground. It builds on a broader ecological approach to the division of labour associated with Durkheim and Everett Hughes by analysing what nurses actually do. This 'organising' work though is not only hidden and unaccounted for but by some estimates approximates to 70 per cent of a nursing role. Hughes, who studied North American nursing extensively during the 1950s, suggested that nurses' 'place in the division of labour is essentially that of doing in a responsible way whatever necessary things are in danger of not being done at all' (Hughes 1984: 308). Hughes' contention however poses a dilemma for professional work since it sits uncomfortably with the notion of jurisdiction with its clearly defined sphere of competence and authority. Nursing work is also subject to tensions flowing from different logics – professional and managerial – in which professional logic assigns primacy to the needs of individuals while the managerial assigns primacy to the efficiency of the organisation in serving population needs. This is not simply a question of numbers but complexity, of patients and the organisational environment in which nurses operate. Allen brings the world of nurses as the system enablers and organisers to light by shining a torch into the 'black hole' which has hitherto eluded us. The key challenge now is to 'translate' that insight into 'articulating' nursing, in its second sense, to the lexicon of nursing labour and measurement of nursing workload. When that has been accomplished the work of this rigorous, richly textured sociological work will have been done.

Anne Marie Rafferty CBE

Preface

Nursing is typically understood, and understands itself, as a care-giving occupation. It is through its relationships with patients that nursing is defined. Yet nursing work extends far beyond direct patient care activities. Across the spectrum of locales in which they are employed, nurses, in numerous ways, support and sustain the delivery and organisation of health services. In recent history, however, this wider work has generally been regarded as at best an adjunct to the core nursing function, and at worse responsible for taking nurses away from their 'real work' with patients. Beyond its identity as the 'other' to care-giving, little is known about this element of nursing practice. For the last 40 years or so, in health policy, academe and public perception, it has remained largely hidden from view. There is, however, a growing recognition that nurses influence service quality as much through their contribution to healthcare systems as through their clinical contact with patients and that understanding nursing work exclusively in terms of the latter is no longer serving the interests of the profession or the public. The aim of this book is to lay the empirical foundations for a reappraisal of the nursing contribution to society by shining a light on this invisible aspect of nurses' work.

Contemporary healthcare systems face very real pressures to improve the safety, quality and efficiency of services in a context of unprecedented financial constraint. Unsurprisingly, then, strengthening service provision is an international policy priority. In this book I argue that nurses are pivotal to healthcare delivery and deploy data derived from observational research on their everyday work in a hospital setting to illustrate this aspect of the nursing role. Drawing together insights from practice-based approaches to work, actor network theory and new institutionalism, I develop a (re)conceptualisation of the social organisation of healthcare and the niche occupied by nursing. Nurses operate in the interstices of health systems, aligning the constellation of actors through which care is delivered, making connections across occupational, departmental and organisational boundaries and mediating the 'needs' of individual patients with the 'needs' of whole populations. This, I argue, entails 'organising work'. My primary objective is to foreground this hitherto neglected dimension of the nursing function, the knowledge and skills that underpin it and those features of healthcare systems that give rise to it. This is necessary to inform nurse education, workforce planning and health services management, which, all too often, are predicated on a faulty understanding of real-life nursing practice. Moreover, as the quality of patient care comes under increased scrutiny in the wake of high profile scandals such as those in the United Kingdom (UK) at Mid Staffordshire National Health Service (NHS) Foundation Trust, this analysis also challenges orthodox understanding of healthcare systems and the role of nurses within them, with important implications for our attempts to improve services and the educational preparation and structure of the nursing workforce.

The fieldwork on which this research is based was carried out during a sabbatical period supported by Cardiff School of Nursing and Midwifery Studies and the data analysis and production of this book were undertaken as part of an Improvement Science Fellowship (2011–2014) funded by The Health Foundation. I am immensely grateful for such investment, enthusiasm and support. Thanks are also due to the senior nurses in the study site who championed the research and the individuals who willingly allowed me to peer over their shoulder while they went about their everyday activities. I am also appreciative of those who assisted with the development of the sampling frame: Sarah Morley, Amanda Monsell, Gillian Knight, Stephen Griffiths, Ann Jones, Alison Evans, Rhian Barnes, Judith Carrier and Elaine Beer. The writing of this book has benefited from critical conversations with Joanna Latimer, Davide Nicolini, Sharon Williams, Maja Korica, Nick Barber and members of the Health Foundation Improvement Science Development Group. Sharon Williams, Christine Ceci, Robert Dingwall and Annette Lankshear generously commented on draft chapters. Responsibility for all shortcomings, however, is entirely my own.

Abbreviations

ANT	Actor Network Theory
BM	Blood Glucose Monitoring
CHC	Continuing Health Care
CIS	Common Information Space
GTN	Glyceryl Trinitrate
GP	General Practitioner
HB	Haemoglobin Level
HCA	Health Care Assistant
IV	Intravenous
NHS	National Health Service
OPA	Outpatient Appointment
PE	Pulmonary Embolism
PMH	Past Medical History
PSAGWB	Patient Status at a Glance White Boards
RCN	Royal College of Nursing
SNP	Specialist Nurse Practitioner
SW	Social Worker
TTH	Tablets to Take Home
UA	Unified Assessment
UK	United Kingdom
UTI	Urinary Tract Infection

1 A figure-ground reversal

Virginia Henderson famously claimed that:

> The unique function of the nurse is to assist the individual, sick or well, in the performance of those activities contributing to health or its recovery (or to peaceful death) that he would perform unaided if he had the necessary strength, will or knowledge.
>
> (Henderson 1966: 15)

Almost 40 years later, after an extensive consultation exercise, the UK Royal College of Nursing (RCN) offered the following definition of the work of the profession:

> The use of clinical judgement in the provision of care to enable people to improve, maintain, or recover health, to cope with health problems, and to achieve the best possible quality of life, whatever their disease or disability, until death.
>
> (Royal College of Nursing 2003: 3)

These quotations illustrate a wider trend spanning the last 40 years, in which nursing's claim to expertise has been expressed exclusively in terms of its care-giving function (Armstrong 1983; May 1992; Allen 2001a). It is through its relationships with patients – whether these are absent, present, good, bad or indifferent – that modern day nursing is defined. The near-universal drive for cost-containment across the international arena has progressively pulled nurses away from this professed metier, but when society becomes concerned about the care of its citizens, it is nurses that are held to account. Yet nurses contribute to service quality in numerous ways which reach far beyond their direct clinical contact with patients. Consider the following:

> It is 11.30 and Maureen has paused at the Nurses' Station to review progress. The ward is the calmest it's been all day. Only a few individuals have yet to be washed and everyone scheduled for theatre this afternoon

is prepared. Sunlight has started to flood into the corridor from the ward areas as one by one the curtains that have enfolded the bed spaces since shortly after breakfast are drawn back. Maureen has just completed processing a newly admitted patient and inserts the various assessment tools, care plans and record forms into the patient's file. She places the medication chart prominently on the Nurses' Station and affixes to it a note requesting that the doctor prescribe night sedation which, she has established, the patient usually takes to help her sleep. Maureen removes a sheet of paper from her pocket, unfolds it and scrutinises the content. It is a list of all patients on the unit; for each a complex set of symbols denotes the current status of their care. Some of these inscriptions are in blue, some in red. The latter is information Maureen has added having attended the ward round earlier. It is her practice to colour code her entries so she can identify readily new developments to be passed on to the person responsible. Several issues now have been attended to: the junior doctor has prescribed medication for the patients going home tomorrow; the discharge letters for the community nursing service are prepared and the receptionist has been instructed to arrange out-patient appointments. Maureen ticks off these items on her sheet and glances at the clock. There is just enough time to telephone the social worker to check the progress of Mr White's home care arrangements before she must leave for the morning meeting to discuss the bed state. All today's discharges are going ahead, but she knows the elective admissions are likely to remain on hold as there are patients in the Emergency Unit who require beds. She hopes she will not have to take patients for whom another service is responsible as the work of organising care for 'outliers' is more difficult, but accepts this is sometimes necessary. Maureen picks up the telephone but quickly returns it to the receiver when she notices that the colorectal nurse specialist has arrived on the unit. She knows she will want an update on Mrs Banner. As they are talking, Maureen takes the opportunity to ask about another patient whose stoma management is interfering with their wound care. The colorectal nurse agrees to change the appliance. Maureen makes a note to this effect on her list. She is now running late for the meeting, so she quickly surveys the bed board and heads off down the corridor. En route she encounters a rather lost-looking junior doctor who inquires, 'Where do you keep purple blood bottles?' 'In there' Maureen replies, pointing to a cupboard on her right and, without breaking her stride, she disappears out of the ward.[1]

This brief episode depicts a typical moment in the day of a nurse responsible for ward coordination and in many ways is wholly unremarkable. Yet it captures many elements of the nursing role that are of interest here: their work in bringing patients into the organisation and mobilising action; their work in maintaining an overview of the current status of individuals' care and communicating this to relevant actors; their work in ensuring all essential activities are carried out and do not interfere with each other; their work in assembling the materials and resources that are required to support conduct; their work in overseeing bed utilisation and their work in facilitating patient transfers. I have called this 'organising work'.

Organising work is that element of the nursing role often referred to as the 'glue' in healthcare systems. Vital as this is for service quality, however, it is largely taken-for-granted, or at least, that is, until things go wrong. Some estimate that this activity counts for more than 70 per cent of the work nurses do (Furaker 2009), yet it rarely features in the profession's public jurisdictional claims and has only ever been studied as a distraction from patient care rather than as a practice in its own right. For example, the RCN develops further the definition quoted above with a description of nursing's six singular characteristics. All centre on the clinical function and, save for a single sentence which acknowledges that '[i]n addition to direct patient care, nursing practice includes management, teaching, and policy and knowledge development' (Royal College of Nursing 2003: 3), nurses' wider contribution to healthcare remains hidden from view. This neglect is mirrored in academia. James (1992) developed the formula 'care = organisation + physical labour + emotional labour' to identify the component parts of care work and to systematically assess how their character and interrelationships varied across different contexts. In recent years, there has been considerable interest in emotional labour as a constituent of nursing work (James 1989; Smith 1992; Bolton 2000, 2001; Smith and Gray 2001; Theodosius 2008) and there is a smaller but emerging field focused on physical labour, including studies of 'body work' (Lawler 1991; Quested and Rudge 2002; Rudge 2009; Cohen 2011) and nurses' technical skills (Sandelowski 2000; Nelson and Gordon 2006; Messman 2008, Pols 2010a, b, 2012; Pols and Willems 2011). Yet 'organisation', understood as the practices through which care is organised, has received relatively little attention. Indeed, while intending for 'organisation' to be read as both a noun and a verb in her formula, James (1992) concentrates her analysis on the former. To draw an analogy with the Gestalt psychology of perception, in nurse education, policy and practice, nurses' organising work is always perceived as the 'ground' to the 'figure' of direct patient care. The famous image depicting both a vase and two profiles of a human face (the Rubin vase) is often used to illustrate the concept of figure-ground. Depending on whether the white or black colour is seen as the figure (forefront) or the ground (background) the brain will interpret the picture as two different images and, according to Gestalt psychological theory, it is impossible to perceive both simultaneously. The figure is what you notice and the ground is everything else. Crucially, the concept of figure-ground depends on the observer and not on the item itself. In the same way that a figure-ground reversal can be used as an intentional visual design technique to create new images, the aim of this book is to place direct patient care in the shadows in order to shine a light on nurses' organising work.

Invisible work

No work is intrinsically visible or invisible; work is made visible through a number of indicators and these change according to the context and the perspectives through which it is viewed (Muller 1999; Star and Strauss 1999). Visible work tends to be equated with formal work that is authorised and documented and thus invisible work is at the heart of politics about what will count as work (Suchman 1995; Hampson and Junor 2005, 2010). Work can be rendered invisible in a number of ways. Some work gets done in invisible places, such as the behind the scenes work of librarians (Nardi and Engeström 1999), the behind the screens work of nurses (Lawler 1991) or the backstage work of food maids (Paterson 1981). Work may be defined as routine when it actually requires skilled problem-solving expertise (Hampson and Junor 2005, 2010). Work can also be done by invisible people. Star and Strauss (1999) reveal how gender, race and class intersect to render domestic workers invisible. They illustrate their argument with the example of an ethnographic study in which the author, an African-American sociologist, passed as a maid and experienced first-hand the processes through which she became progressively 'unseeable' by her employers (Rollins 1985). Hart (1991) makes similar observations in her study of hospital domestics. In the reverse of this scenario, the worker can be visible, but the work can be relegated to the background. 'If one looked, one *could* literally see the work being done – but the taken for granted status means that it is functionally invisible' (Star and Strauss 1999: 20 original emphasis).

The premise that we have special authority in relation to our own knowledge and expertise suggests that we should have the ability to shape not only how we work, but also how that work is perceived (Suchman 1995). Yet workers themselves are not always aware of their contribution to an overall activity (Nardi and Engeström 1999), may not have a language with which to describe certain tacit skills or the confidence with which to assert their claims. Moreover, studies have shown that some types of work are more likely to be invisible than others. Feminist scholars have drawn attention to the invisible work of women who are often employed in service sector posts, poorly remunerated because their role is believed to rest on natural attributes rather than workplace skills. It is also the case that the better the work is done the less visible it is to those who benefit from it (Suchman 1995). In their public jurisdictional claims occupations elect to foreground certain activities over others. Some work may remain invisible therefore because it creates strains with an occupational identity (Hughes 1984).

Visibility and invisibility are not inherently good or bad. In 1968 200 female sewing machinists famously stopped production at the Ford Motor Company in Dagenham when they went on strike following a re-grading exercise in which their work was classified as 'unskilled' whereas comparable work done by men was classified as 'semi-skilled'. The strike is widely regarded as prompting the passing of the UK Equal Pay Act in 1970. Greater visibility can also result in increased control and surveillance, however. Bowker *et al.* (2001) analyse an attempt by nurses from the University of Iowa to categorise nursing practice and trace the delicate balancing act this entailed whereby nurses struggled to gain formal recognition for their work while simultaneously maintaining areas of discretion. Beyond the direct consequences for workers, the visibility–invisibility of work has implications for organisations. A number of studies have shown that technology implementation and/or workplace restructuring advanced on the basis of only work that is visible can run into difficulties. For example, Westerberg (1999) studied home care in Sweden and describes how workers operated with a formal visible vertical organisational structure and informal horizontal social networks. Both were critical to the management of the work and served important functions that ensured citizens received high quality home care. Despite its potential to augment the informal networks, however, a new computer system was designed to support only the formal structure. In the Danish public sector, Stroebaek (2013) highlights the importance of coffee breaks in sustaining communities of coping that enabled workers to deal with emotionally demanding jobs, through sharing cases and exchanging professional opinions as well as expressing personal frustrations. Stroebaek argues that coffee breaks should not be considered as the 'waste fabric' of productivity, but an important part of the work. Similarly, in the inexorable drive for efficiency, organisations increasingly find it necessary to slim down and this may involve judgements about the necessity of the work being done, the numbers of staff required or the mix of skills involved. If such decisions are based on a flawed understanding of the work, the consequences can be serious.

Nursing work has many features that make visibility problematic. It is gendered work and thus falls into that category of work that is often assumed to rest on the natural talents of women. It is also body work (Twigg *et al.* 2011) which requires the transgression of normal social boundaries (Lawler 1991); so it is work that cannot be talked about. The work of nurses is also extraordinarily diverse and another factor which has contributed to its invisibility – or at least to the invisibility of certain elements – is the challenge the profession has faced in developing a conceptual frame and professional identity which encapsulates the diverse range of activities that nurses do (Beardshaw and Robinson 1990). Fields of work are forever changing too – none more so than healthcare – and this affects the visibility or invisibility of work and the organisational consequences of this relationship. In the next section I trace the shifting contours of healthcare and its implications for nursing and the visibility of its work.

Nursing in the twenty-first century

The evolution of modern healthcare systems is having a profound effect on the work of nurses. In the UK over the last 20–30 years, structural, technical, demographic and policy changes have impacted on the context, content and pace of nursing practice. Hospital nurses have experienced increased devolution of managerial responsibility and are expected to process faster more acutely ill patients and simultaneously contain service costs (Annandale 1996; Latimer 2000). Community nurses have faced similar pressures (Charles-Jones *et al.* 2003) and must respond to the challenges presented by a rebalancing of secondary and community care provision in support of a growing number of frail older people. Changes in skill-mix following the Project 2000 reforms of nurse education (UKCC 1987) have compelled qualified nurses to devise new ways of working with support staff, while policies for the preparation of junior doctors (Allen 1997) and the evolution of medical technologies (Tjora 2000; Charles-Jones *et al.* 2003; Mort *et al.* 2004) create the impetus for the delegation of new tasks. Wider democratic impulses have precipitated a redistribution of work across the lay-professional interface (Allen and Pilnick 2005) requiring nurses to practice in partnership with patients and families (Allen 2000a, b) and deliver user-centred services. At the same time, and in common with other health and social care providers, nurses' work is subject to growing standardisation and external scrutiny through new systems of clinical governance and quality improvement (Berg 1997; Power 1997; Dent 1999; Purkis 2001; Purkis and Bjornsdottir 2006; Crawford and Brown 2008; Traynor 2009; Allen 2010a, b; Bevan 2010; Morrow *et al.* 2012).

Against this background, a body of critical policy commentary has emerged indicating that the traditional nursing mandate, with its exclusive focus on care-giving, is no longer serving the profession or the public (Lawson 1996; Horton 1997; Dingwall and Allen 2001; Glen 2004; Maben and Griffiths 2008). This has been buttressed by growing societal unease about the quality of nursing care, most recently brought to a head by a number of high-profile scandals, such as that centred on Mid-Staffordshire NHS Foundation Trust which reported widespread shortcomings in fundamental clinical standards (House of Commons 2010, 2013) and St George's Hospital, Tooting, in which a 22-year-old patient died from dehydration (Davies 2012). Professional mandates have an important role in making work publically visible, transmitting occupational culture and defining group membership (Whittaker and Olesen 1964; Gabriel 1993). They are also important in encouraging members to strive for their principles when there is a strain towards compromise in the work setting (James 1992). If the gap between professional ideals and reality becomes too wide, however, mandates can become dysfunctional (Becker 1970). For many, this mismatch can result in alienation from work, in a classic Marxist sense, leading to burn-out, withdrawal from employment or diminished commitment reflected in indifferent standards of care (Dingwall and Allen 2001; Maben *et al.* 2006). Critically, for current purposes, not only does such misalignment distort expectations for practice, it does not reflect what nurses actually do in practice, and thus prevents the profession from realising its potential.

All too often prescriptions for nursing have arisen from armchair theorising about what nurses *should* do rather than research into what they *actually* do and an understanding of how this role function is shaped by the contexts in which they work. Hospital nursing is an organisationally-embedded occupation, having emerged in parallel with the growth of the modern healthcare system, but it has tended to be understood through the lens of a prototypical profession predicated on an untrammelled one-to-one relationship with clients. For example, Celia Davies (1995) described nurses' 'professional predicament' in terms of the 'polo mint problem'. The polo mint is a confection characterised by a hole at its centre, and the analogy is intended to signify the effect created by all the tasks required to support the healthcare system which, according to Davies, are responsible for pulling nursing away from its core work with patients thereby creating a gap through which the care-giving function is lost.

Yet the nursing role has always included a wide range of background activities which do not entail direct care delivery. In her 'Notes on Nursing', Nightingale asserted that:

> Bad sanitary, bad architectural, and bad administrative arrangements often make it impossible to nurse. But the art of nursing ought to include such arrangements as alone make what I understand by nursing, possible.
>
> (Nightingale 1860/1969: 8)

For Nightingale, then, 'care' entailed being responsible for creating the environments that foster healing and health. The sociologist Everett Hughes, who studied North American nursing extensively during the 1950s, suggested that nurses' 'place in the division of labour is essentially that of doing in a responsible way whatever necessary things are in danger of not being done at all' (Hughes 1984: 308) and, in my own review of 54 ethnographic studies of nursing work spanning six countries published between 1993 and 2003, I identified eight bundles of tasks undertaken by nurses which contributed to healthcare delivery that did not entail direct contact with patients (Allen 2004, 2007). Despite widespread acknowledgement of its pervasiveness, however, to the best of my knowledge, the non-care-giving element of the nursing function has never been studied in its own right, and has tended to be described through negative metaphors. Thus, Davies refers to nurses' organisational contribution as 'adjunct work' and Mauksch (1966) compared nursing work to the network of dough which remains on the work surface after all the individual cookies have been cut out:

> We are reminded of a sheet of rolled-out dough from which the housewife has cut many cookies, which, on an aluminium sheet, are baking in the oven. What is left on the kitchen table is a network of dough which still suggests the entire original scope and area of the

previously cut solid surface. Somehow, nursing is reminiscent of the pattern which remains after the cookies have been cut.

(Mauksch 1966: 124)

To a considerable extent, nurses' organising work is the 'dirty work' of the profession. Hughes (1984) coined this term to refer to work that posed a threat to an occupation's identity and in nursing, much ink has been spilt in academe on the question of how nursing practice can be brought back into alignment with the profession's ideals. In the context of growing concerns about deteriorating standards of basic care, arguments about the negative effects of 'non-clinical' activities on the 'real work' of nurses undoubtedly have credence. For example, they are implicit in recent quality improvement interventions, like the Productive Ward series, designed to rationalise healthcare delivery (Morrow *et al.* 2012). With their claims to 'release time to care', such initiatives appeal to the contemporary nursing mandate and resonate strongly with wider policy concerns about service quality. Indeed, one might aver that the effectiveness of such rhetorical strategies is one reason for the widespread diffusion of the Productive Ward and its derivatives. But they also presuppose that nurses' 'non-patient' work is not a legitimate use of their skills or, at the very least, that it claims more of their time than is desirable. But where is the evidence to substantiate these assumptions? In industrial contexts improvement models are based on the axiom that organisations first understand their production process. All too often in their application to healthcare, however, tools and techniques are introduced to substitute for an aspect of the work which, because of its invisibility, is poorly understood.

Stimulated by the sense that the profession had lost its way, in 2008 the UK National Nursing Research Unit produced a report on the role of nurses in society (Maben and Griffiths 2008). Its recommendations were designed to restore confidence in nursing, define what the public and nurses want and identify a series of measures to secure a step change in the quality of care. A new model of professionalism is proposed which entails recasting the nursing role beyond the care of patients to include the contribution they make to their organisations and the whole health service. The need for such work is increasingly evident as healthcare leaders across the world reflect on how best to ensure the quality and safety of patient care. In this book I begin to lay the foundations for such a transition by developing a new, empirically derived, conceptualisation of a critical element of nursing practice.

Studying nurses' organising work

Research on nursing work often is predicated on essentialist conceptions about the nursing function. Thus it is supposed that nursing has necessary properties, which logically precede the situated practices which instantiate nursing work and, as we have seen, much nursing research is concerned with addressing the mismatch between these assumptions and the constraints of the practice setting. I take a different approach. I draw on ecological approaches to the division of labour and practice-based theories and my concern is with studying the work that nurses actually do and the system features which give rise to it.

Ecological thinking can be traced back to the French sociologist Durkheim (1933), through the work of Everett Hughes (Hughes 1951, 1984; Hughes *et al*. 1958), Eliot Freidson (1976) and most recently Andrew Abbott (1988). It is an approach which invites us to think about the world of work as a dynamic social system and to study the connections between social groups and institutions and their interdependence in a wider field of action. For these theorists, the system of work is forever changing in response to economic, technological and social factors which reshape occupations. New tasks emerge or are redistributed to other occupational groups, others disappear completely. Activities that were once the work of formal waged occupations may be passed to the unwaged sector. The boundaries between different occupations expand and contract in an ongoing evolutionary process in which new occupations materialise, others fuse and some may decline or vanish entirely (Dingwall 1983; Allen 2001a).

Nursing tends to be at the forefront of wider changes in healthcare owing to its intimate connection to health service organisations and because of its location in the division of labour in which it devolves work to lower grades on the one hand, and receives delegated tasks from medicine and management on the other. While recent literature on the impact of healthcare reforms written from a nursing perspective frequently laments that nurses are being taken away from their true vocation by such wider external social forces (Dingwall and Allen 2001), from a sociological perspective, evolution and change is an inevitable feature of all systems of work and thus should be expected. As Hughes (1984: 286) has argued, an occupation, in essence, is not some particular set of functions: 'it is the part of an individual in any on-going system of activities.' Sociologically speaking, then, the division of labour is only incidentally technical. It consists not of intrinsic skills or of mechanical or mental operations, but of the actual allocation of functions to persons, that is, their role within a sphere of action. While it may be possible for an occupation to be predicated on one activity in a narrow technical sense, they are more typically comprised of a number or a 'bundle' of practices. Certain of these may be grouped together because they involve similar skills, others because they can be conveniently done in one place, or because taken alone they do not occupy a worker's full time, and some because they are seen to be natural parts of a certain role. Hughes (1984) suggests that it is possible to analyse occupations according to the domination of technical as against role factors in determining the combinations of practices. As an organisationally-embedded profession, nursing is a good example of an occupation in which role factors have been most significant in shaping its overall function. Indeed, over its history, nursing has proven to be extremely adaptable and ready to absorb changes in job content, assimilating many diverse responsibilities. But this has also led periodically to the kinds of crises of occupational identity with which the profession is currently wrestling (Carpenter 1977).

In studying nurses' organising work I have drawn on a broad family of theories which share a number of conceptual similarities and which are increasingly understood as practice-based approaches (Nicolini 2012). The origins of this way of thinking can be traced through praxeology (Bourdieu 1977, 1990), ethnomethodology (Garfinkel 1967), structuration (Giddens 1984) and activity theory (Engeström *et al.* 2002; Engeström 2008). They share several broad orientations in common (Nicolini 2012).

First, they conceive of social phenomena as created through human agency and continuously in process. Apparently durable social structures such as gender or organisation are understood as verbs rather than nouns, that is, as an ongoing practical accomplishment. Of interest, then, are the processes through which this is achieved. Garfinkel (1967), in a famous ethnomethodological example, traces the unfolding practices through which Agnes, a transsexual, brought off the task of passing as a normal woman and in my own work I have revealed how nurses' jurisdictional boundaries are actively constructed in practice rather than taken as given (Allen 2001a, b).

Second, practices are conceptualised as bodily activities made possible by an array of resources. Practice theories emphasise that human subjects do not relate to the world directly; activity is always mediated by artefacts of some kind. In healthcare, these may be material artefacts such as surgical instruments, protocols or paper-based forms, or psychological artefacts such as heuristics, medical concepts, categories and methods. Artefacts embody diverse assumptions or 'scripts' and are structured in different ways and these 'affordances' (Hutchby 2001) shape the possibilities for action. Indeed artefacts do not just support human endeavour, they transform the nature of the task. Thus, of particular interest is the relationship between tools and human action and how practice is distributed between them. Berg's work on the uses of the medical record and related health information technologies is a good example of this kind of sensitivity (Berg 1996, 1997, 1998, 1999).

Third, a practice-based approach always leaves space for human creativity and initiative. Performing a practice is neither mindless repetition nor complete invention (Nicolini 2012); practice must be understood as emerging from dynamic interactions with the material and social world as people find solutions to their problems. Work is unpredictable, ill structured or emergent (often all of these) and people need creative processes to find solutions to their problems (Suchman 1987). Thus, practice theories highlight how people make sense of their circumstances, but eschew sensemaking as some kind of private mental process, locating it instead in the material and discursive activities of members (Weick 1995).

Fourth, practice-based approaches underline the importance of power. Practices serve certain interests and they do this through the relationships that are created through networks of practices and how these fit into a given context and its distribution of power and privileges (Ortner 1984). So, in studying nursing, it is important to ask about the constraints that are placed on their organising work as well as the consequences of these practices for others. Practices may always be contested which maintains them in a continuous state of change and they are located in historical and material conditions so, in principle at least, if practices were different then the world would be a different place (Ortner 1984). Echoing the Weberian distinction between 'power' and 'authority' (Gerth and Mills 1946), I will argue that at one level nursing is powerfully placed through its practices to shape the quality of care patients receive. At another level, they face the challenge of having these practices treated as legitimate.

Finally, adopting a practice perspective transforms how we comprehend knowledge. Thus, knowledge is understood as the capacity to undertake a social and material activity, it is a 'set of practical methods acquired through learning, inscribed in objects, embodied, and only partially articulated in discourse' (Nicolini 2012: 5). Becoming a contributor to a particular field of practice entails learning how to act and how to speak, but also what to feel, what to expect and what things mean. As Bourdieu (2000) has observed, different fields in social life engender a certain set of social relations in which actors engage in their everyday practice. Through this practice they will develop a certain disposition (lasting, acquired schemes of perception, thought and activity) for social action, that foster a tendency to act in a particular way, which he termed 'habitus'. This has important implications for how we understand nurses' organising work and the implications this has for education and professional development.

In addition to practice-based approaches, I have also drawn on insights from actor network theory (ANT). ANT has its origins in studies of the networks of interdependent social practices that constitute work in science and technology and arises from the scholarship of Michel Callon (1986) and Bruno Latour (1991, 1998, 2005). John Law (1992) has extended this model for the whole of sociology. ANT is a complex field and there has been much discussion about its underlying precepts, its uses and abuses and whether it is actually a theory (Law and Hassard 1999). There is no need to enter into these debates here. The value of ANT in complementing a practice-based approach is that it affords an analytic sensitivity to the *relationships* between the heterogeneous elements comprising a field of practice and a language with which to describe these.

The assertion that both human and non-human actors are equally actants within a network is a central contribution of ANT to this field. While 'actors' are normally understood as conscious beings, actants comprise all sorts of autonomous figures which make up our world and are endowed with the ability to act (people, concepts, text, material objects, statements and artefacts). For scholars with an interest in fields of work, this orientation opens up the possibility of thinking about the allocation of functions between human and non-human actors. For example, in recent years healthcare has witnessed a proliferation of artefacts designed to support the coordination of work: care pathways, checklists and algorithms. ANT invites analysis of the actions these are being asked to fulfil and the implications this has for the users of the tool, processes that are termed delegation and prescription respectively (Latour 1998). Such divisions are not fixed: they are open to negotiation and change – so non-humans gain or lose attributes – and so too do people (Law 1992).

Within ANT, all social phenomena are analysed as actor-networks. However, the use of the term network should not be confused with more technical applications of this notion:

> We are not primarily concerned with mapping interactions between individuals [...] we are concerned to map the way in which they [actors] define and distribute roles, and mobilize or invent others to play those roles.
>
> (Law and Callon 1988: 285, cited by Cressman 2009)

Thus, actor-networks are shifting systems of alliances of heterogeneous elements.

Networks are potentially transient, and have to be actively performed, made and remade, in order to retain their stability. Moreover, they are not intrinsically coherent, and may contain conflicts and disagreements. Accordingly, a prevailing interest in ANT has been with how relations within a network stay in place or how it is that patterns or links remain stable. Actors within a network are understood to take the shape that they do because of their relations with each other and they derive their identity from their interaction with others (Cressman 2009). Any form of social ordering is the effect of the associations within a heterogeneous network; for ANT there are no causes, just effects. ANT is concerned with how networks gain coherence and consistency (stabilisation).

'Translation' is the broad term used within ANT for the processes by which network elements are held together, through the alignment of goals and concerns, or by keeping contradictory elements apart. Translation has both a geometric and a semiotic meaning: it refers to the movement of an entity in space and time, as well as its translation from one context to another. The latter has parallels with the translation from one language to another, with the necessary transformation of meaning this implies (Gherardi and Nicolini 2005). Although ANT does not usually explain why or how a network takes the form that it does, it provides a method and a lens for looking at the world so the relational ties within a network can be explored.

> [Translation is] the process of making connections, of forging a passage between two domains, or simply establishing communication. [It is] an

act of invention brought about through combination and mixing of varied elements.

(Brown 2002: 3–6, quoted by Cressman 2009)

The process of translation has three main elements and numerous actors within a network may be involved in a different process of translation. The first moment of translation is referred to as 'problematisation' in which an actor defines the activities of other actors which are consistent with its own interests and establishes itself as functionally indispensible. The second moment is known as 'interessement', and involves the process of convincing other actors to accept the definition of the focal actor. 'Enrolment' refers to the moment when another actor accepts these interests as defined.

For analytic purposes it is useful to focus on a single actor, and consider translational processes from its vantage point. So, for example, in this book healthcare is considered from the stance of nursing. Nurses, I argue, may be considered 'obligatory passage points' in healthcare organisations. Obligatory passage points are focal actors in an actor network that shape and mobilise the network and through which all others must pass. Described by some as the network's panopticon (Dear and Flusty 2002), an obligatory passage point is a privileged location which can see and act at a distance and 'have control over all transactions between the local and global networks' (Law and Callon 1994: 31).

In studying the elements of a network, ANT distinguishes between intermediaries and mediators. Intermediaries are entities which make no difference to the phenomena of interest whereas mediators multiply difference and so should be the object of study. They are the means for bringing together the various heterogeneous entities in a network thereby constructing the form and the substance of the relations set up between them. Simplified networks are those which are sufficiently stabilised to become black-boxed, such that the complex socio-material relationships through which they are constituted are rendered invisible. The process by which networks become black-boxed is referred to as 'punctualisation' (Crawford 2004): 'the process of punctualization thus converts an entire network into a single point or node in another network' (Callon 1991: 153). From an ANT perspective, everything is both an actor and a network; it depends on the perspective.

ANT also usefully offers an approach to the consideration of power and can be considered a theory of the mechanisms of power, that is, the stabilisation and reproduction of some interactions over others. Rather than power as a possession, power may be understood as persuasion and is generated in a relational and distributed manner as a consequence of ordering struggles.

Although originating from singular theoretical traditions, taken together this family of approaches affords a useful orienting framework through which to study and articulate nurses' organising work. Specific concepts will be explored in greater detail as they are introduced into the analysis.

The data

The research on which this book is based was undertaken at a large University Health Board in Wales, referred to here by the pseudonym: Parklands. Between March and August 2011 I shadowed 40 hospital nurses working in adult care settings with the aim of better understanding 'organising work'. My interest was in the functions of nurses in frontline clinically-oriented roles, rather than formal management posts. Following Spradley (1980), my focus was on what nurses did, the tools they used and what these practices revealed about what they know. The primary sources of data were non-participant observation, informal qualitative interviews, and the analysis of documents and material artefacts. Individuals were shadowed while they worked and this was combined with observations of the wider environment in order to understand the system factors that gave rise to their practice. On average 8 hours of fieldwork was undertaken with each study participant, arranged to take into account the nature of the role and individuals' capacity to carry out their work with an ethnographer looking over their shoulder. Observational data were supplemented by informal interviews which explored participants' work, its meaning and the skills and knowledge involved. The data generated were recorded in a spiral-bound jotter as low-inference field notes and word processed at the earliest opportunity. Research ethics approval was granted by the Cardiff School of Nursing and Midwifery Studies Research Ethics Committee.

The selection of study participants was informed by an expert reference group drawn from nurse education, research, service and policy. A typology of environments identified as likely to be consequential for nursing practice was developed in order to purposively select an initial maximum variation sample of role formats so as to capture the full spectrum of nurses' organising work. Exhaustive coverage of all fields or the full nursing function was not intended; rather, the purpose was to identify those posts which would be most perspicacious given the research aims. Twelve roles were selected initially, with others subsequently added as a result of the concurrent analysis. The final sample comprised service-based rotating roles (undertaken by different team members periodically) and posts occupied by individuals on a permanent basis. The sample was almost exclusively female; only two participants were male. I shadowed several participants working in specialist nursing roles, including the acute pain management and colorectal nurses whose work combined clinical and organisational elements. I spent time, too, with nurses who worked in roles that incorporated a gate-keeping function, such as the cardiac coordinator, the stroke coordinator and the anaesthetic pre-assessment nurses, and others, such as the rehabilitation specialist nurse and the discharge liaison nurses, whose primary responsibilities related to the negotiation of interfaces to secure transfers of care. The work of nurses in service-based coordinator roles was also observed. In areas where throughput was rapid – such as the Emergency

Unit, the Medical and Surgical Assessment Units and the Short-Stay Surgical Unit – their function was to manage patient flows and bed utilisation, the demands of which were all-consuming. There were coordinators in the intensive care areas too. I shadowed the nurses working in this capacity in the general and cardiac intensive care units. Here the role combined organising the work of the department, overseeing the effective deployment of staff and supervision of junior nurses. In the general ward areas, the nurses working in this capacity liaised with the multitude of specialists that attended to patients, handled transfers of care and orchestrated discharge arrangements. It is important to stress, however, that this was not a study of nursing roles as such; a practice-based approach takes practices as the unit of analysis rather than the practitioners, accordingly my focus was on the organising component of the nursing function.

The hallmark of good ethnographic field relations is the successful management of a marginal status. Methods textbooks underline the importance of developing an affinity with participants while retaining the necessary intellectual distance for the research. Compared to conventional ethnographic research, the time spent with individuals in this study was limited. This made for extremely intense fieldwork where the challenge was not that of maintaining marginality, but of rapidly developing a relationship with research participants in order to gain insights into their social worlds. On the whole, despite the relatively short time I spent with them, this was successfully achieved and the nurses did not seem guarded in their conversations with me or appear to modify their behaviour because of my presence.

Data generation and analysis proceeded concurrently. Ideas prompted in the course of writing up field notes were embedded in the ethnographic record, but differentiated from the rest of the text. In addition, at the end of each observational episode I delineated my thoughts on the research process. These included themes that had arisen, gaps in understanding, issues to pursue and broader lines of inquiry related to the emerging findings. I routinely shared my observations and interpretations with the individuals I shadowed to ensure I had not overlooked anything they considered to be important or misunderstood an aspect of their role. These conversations were a constructive check on the emerging analysis. Presenting the research at the senior nurses' meeting after five months of fieldwork was an additional valuable opportunity to test whether my observations made sense from their perspective. Throughout the study, I periodically reviewed the whole data set, drawing out similarities across, and differences between roles, so as to assemble the findings into broad themes. Once fieldwork had ended, all data were entered into computer assisted qualitative data analysis software: Atlas/ti. The program permits the electronic tagging (coding) of data extracts to support data management. An initial descriptive coding frame was devised to facilitate data retrieval and refined in accordance with the emerging analysis. Ideas generated inductively from the data were then considered in the light of relevant literatures.

The original sample included community nurses and it was my intention to take account of their work in the analysis. However, as this progressed, I realised that organising work and organisational context are closely intertwined and understanding the nursing function and the factors that facilitate and inhibit nursing practice required an exploration of this relationship. Accordingly, I have elected to concentrate on the work of hospital nurses, partly because my data are inadequate for the purposes of examining community nurses' organising work in sufficient depth and partly because it would be impossible to do justice to both in a single book. My hope is that the analysis presented here will lay the foundations for further research in the community context. Safeguarding the quality of hospital care is a pressing concern, but so too is the need for new models of community services to support those living with long-term physical and psychological conditions and the growing number of frail older people. Nurses are central to each of these interrelated policy priorities.

Nursing work and the modern hospital

Hospitals are built, staffed and equipped for treatment of the sick and injured. The last 40 years has witnessed a transformation in hospital care across the developed world. There has been a steady decline in the number of in-patient beds, more than matched by faster throughput and increased rates of hospitalisation (Armstrong 1998). Average length of stay has fallen substantially since 1980, typically by about 50 per cent. Advances in medical science have enabled more active treatment of people with co-morbidities and thus patients in hospital require more demanding management (Aiken *et al*. 2012). Hospitals are profoundly complex organisations; technologically rich and knowledge-intensive, they are comprised of multiple units and departments and characterised by a highly specialised division of labour. There is a growing recognition that as healthcare work becomes increasingly concentrated and multifacted, excellent patient care depends not on individual brilliance but on the coordination of activity to ensure that the appropriate configuration of actors – actions, technology, expertise, materials – are in place to support individual needs. This requires organising work. As the pressure in the acute sector increases to ensure high quality care that is safe while simultaneously accelerating patient throughput, the need for this grows exponentially.

The delivery and organisation of healthcare is challenging. Recent decades have witnessed an explosion of technologies that draw on systems engineering and management science in order to rationalise service processes and work activity. Nurses have contributed to these developments, emerging as the lead profession in the implementation of formal tools such as local protocols and integrated care pathways (McDonald and Harrison 2004; Allen 2009, 2010a, b). Yet, healthcare work often defies such standardisation and control. Individual disease processes can be unpredictable and many patients have co-morbidities and multifarious needs which are a poor fit with standardised models. Even in those cases where alignment with a formal plan is possible, the care of individuals takes place in organisations responsible for clinical populations, and as such, patients are in competition with each other for access to services, facilities and the time and attention of health professionals. Sometimes this can be managed systematically through formal systems of triage and scheduling, but often not; hospitals are less able to control their inputs than can other industries. It is also the case that despite its ever-increasing technical sophistication, healthcare is ineluctably 'people work'; patients and their families not only have a view of the 'production' process, they are also co-producers and, whereas in industrial contexts production and consumption are separated, in healthcare they are simultaneous activities (Osborne *et al.* 2012; Radnor and Osborne 2013). Thus, much of healthcare is less like a closely controlled production line and rather more like the work of Mark Twain's celebrated Mississippi River pilot:

> [T]he river was tricky, changed its course slightly from day-to-day, so even an experienced, but inattentive pilot could run into grave difficulties; worse yet, sometimes the river drastically shifted in its bed for some miles into a new course.
>
> (Strauss *et al.* 1985: 19–20)

This disconnection between the messy everyday reality of much of healthcare work and the proliferation of rationalising techniques and technologies derived from management science may be understood by drawing on insights from new institutionalism. New institutionalism is a theory that attends to the deeper and more resilient aspects of social structure – religion, family, and capitalism, for instance – and has its origins in the work of a number of classical theorists, such as Weber, Parsons and Marx. It takes as its focal interest the processes through which social structures, including schemas, norms, rules and routines, become authoritative guidelines for behaviour (Scott 2005). New institutional theory is relevant to all aspects of social life, but there is a significant body of scholarship and empirical work, which emerged in the 1980s, that has applied these ideas to organisations.

According to new institutional theory, organisations are specialised subsystems of large societal structures, and in order to survive they need not only to be successful economically they must also establish legitimacy. New institutionalism argues that to make a legitimate claim on scarce resources the goals organisations pursue should be congruent with wider societal values. In this context, legitimacy can be understood as 'a generalized perception or assumption that the actions of an entity are desirable, proper, or appropriate within some socially constructed system of norms, values, beliefs, and definitions' (Suchman 1995: 574).

These insights were taken up by Meyer and Rowan (1977) who were the first to call attention to how organisations seek legitimacy and support by incorporating structures and procedures that match widely accepted cultural models. As a consequence, they argue, much that happens in organisations stems not from the demands of the work, but from symbols, beliefs and rituals. According to Meyer and Rowan modern societies are dominated by norms of rationality which play a causal role in the creation of formal organisations, providing the templates for their design. They argue that many aspects of formal structure are driven less by competition or the need for efficiency, rather, they are highly institutionalised myths depicting the appropriate means for the attainment of desirable ends.

> By designing a formal structure that adheres to the prescription myths in the institutional environment, an organization demonstrates that it is acting on collectively valued purposes in a proper and adequate manner [...]. The incorporation of institutionalized elements provides an account (Scott and Lyman 1968) of its activities that protects the organization from having its conduct questioned. The organization becomes, in a word, legitimate. [...] The labels of the organization chart as well as the vocabulary used to delineate organizational goals, procedures, and policies are analogous to the vocabularies of motive used to account for the activities of individuals (Mills 1940; Blum and McHugh 1971). Just as jealously, anger, altruism, and love are myths that interpret and explain the actions of individuals, the myths of doctors, of accountants, or of the assembly line explain organizational activities. [...]. Vocabularies of structure which are isomorphic with institutional rules provide prudent, rational, and legitimate accounts. Organizations described in legitimated vocabularies are assumed to be oriented to collectively defined, and often collectively mandated, ends.
>
> (Meyer and Rowan 1977: 349)

Building on this work, DiMaggio and Powell (1983) introduced the notion of an organisational field to denote the proximal institutional environment in which organisations operate and which generates distinctive cultural pressures about the appropriate ways of acting that transcend any single organisation's purposive control (Suchman 1995). This is why, within a given domain, there is a tendency for organisations to increasingly resemble one another – referred to by DiMaggio and Powell (1983) as isomorphism – even if they do not become more efficient. While early adopters of organisational innovation are driven by the desire to improve performance, over time new practices become 'infused with value beyond the technical requirements of the task at hand' (Selznick 1957: 17, cited by DiMaggio and Powell 1983).

According to DiMaggio and Powell (1983), there are three types of isomorphic process. 'Coercive isomorphism' arises from political influence and can be a direct response to a government mandate. 'Mimetic isomorphism' arises from standard responses to uncertainty; thus when technologies are poorly understood or the environment is ambiguous, organisations model themselves on others. A third source of isomorphism is 'normative' and this stems primarily from professionalisation and the need for occupations to establish a basis for autonomy. Institutional environments are not unitary, however, they often contain varied systems of norms, values and beliefs about the appropriate ways of behaving – what some have termed institutional logics (Freidland and Alford 1991). Thus, in healthcare, professional and managerial institutions coexist as divergent or competing models for organising action (Kitchener 2002; Scott 2004).

The bases of legitimacy are not static. For example, modern societies place greater emphasis on corporate and state influences whereas earlier societies placed greater emphasis on family and religion. Over the last 30 years the prominence of neoliberal logics has been found in multiple studies in various contexts (Thorton and Ocasio 2008) and while historically healthcare organisations gained legitimacy from professional logics, more recently they have been penetrated by market and managerial logics which has had a profound effect on their formal structures. More so than most organisations, hospitals have traditionally attempted to separate and insulate the sphere of technical tasks under the jurisdiction of medical staff from administrative tasks under the control of managers (Ruef and Scott 1998). In recent years, however, this has become increasingly unsustainable. In the wake of high profile scandals about the quality and safety of care, healthcare systems are confronted by a growing crisis of legitimacy and as neoliberalism increasingly infuses all aspects of society, organisations have increasingly appealed to these logics in order to secure legitimacy. The guidelines, checklists and protocols which have propagated in healthcare over the past three decades can be understood as an attempt to signal to the outside world that the organisation takes its internal procedures seriously and is making a good faith effort to achieve valued ends. We might think of this as procedural legitimacy (Scott 1977, cited by Suchman 1995).

According to Meyer and Rowan (1977: 355), 'formal structures that celebrate institutionalized myths differ from structures that act efficiently' and they suggest that the way in which organisations accommodate these tensions is by routinely decoupling formal structures produced in response to institutional demands from technical work processes. This formulation has not been received uncritically, however. While it has long been recognised that organisations were often quite loosely coupled, the notion of decoupling seemed to imply for many connotations of deception or ceremonial compliance which sat uneasily with the empirical experiences of a number of scholars (Scott 2005). Moreover, what this image of organisations does not allow for, is situations, as is currently the case in healthcare, in which institutional forces have promoted the intrusion of management control into technical operations via a whole range of clinical governance and rationalising technologies such that these are entangled and must be accommodated in everyday practice. Thus decoupling may not be as absolute as Meyer and Rowan propose. Scott and Meyer (1983) developed an intermediate position in which it is argued that technical performance pressures are not necessarily opposed but somewhat orthogonal to institutional forces. Nevertheless, an enduring truth associated with the original argument is that modern organisational structures are a product not only of coordinative demands imposed by complex technologies but also of rationalised norms legitimating adoption of appropriate models.

In addition to thinking about hospital organisations through the insights offered by new institutionalism, a further central organising concept of this book is the notion of a 'care trajectory'. This is based on Strauss *et al.*'s (1985) 'illness trajectory' concept, developed as a way of studying the social organisation of healthcare work in the face of its growing complexity. In its original formulation, the term refers 'not only to the physiological unfolding of a patient's disease but to the total *organization of work* done over that course, plus the *impact* on those involved with that work and its organization' (1985: 8, original emphasis). Dominant approaches to organisational analysis at the time emphasised stable structures, but in marked contrast, Strauss *et al.* (1985) conceptualised healthcare organisations as *negotiated orders*, emergent and continuously in process. For my purposes, the illness trajectory concept is preferable to the more commonly used contemporary notion of patient pathway as it avoids the growing association of this latter term in policy and practice with a planned course of action. Yet, the notion of an '*illness* trajectory' is not entirely satisfactory either. It is implicitly predicated on a medical model and, with its emphasis on physiological processes, is a rather outdated conceptualisation given that much of contemporary healthcare work is concerned not just with disease management, but also patients' wider requirement for ongoing care and support. So it makes more sense to talk about a '*care* trajectory' which we might think of as referring to the unfolding of a patient's health and social care needs, the total organisation of work carried out over its course and the impact on those involved with that work and its organisation (Allen *et al.* 2004).

From a practice-based perspective, a care trajectory can be conceptualised as an activity system. This is the basic unit of analysis in activity theory and it refers to the constellation of interrelated practices and artefacts oriented towards a shared object, in this case, the patient. Activities are not regarded as belonging to an individual but are part of a collective endeavour with an associated division of labour, tools, artefacts, norms, rules and conventions. Collaboration is achieved by distributing the goals between different actors who align their actions according to the objective of the overall activity. According to activity theory, three characteristics define the object of all practices (Nicolini 2012).

First, the object is partly given, but partly emergent. Thus the object is constructed and negotiated by the community that gathers around it. Patient care is marked by much uncertainty, ambiguity and unexpected contingencies and as a consequence the question of 'what are we here for?' is never resolved once and for all, but must be worked out as part of the ongoing work activity. Indeed, while healthcare providers may agree on their higher order purpose, at the level of everyday practice they often operate with different motivations and objectives (Allen *et al.* 2004). Effective working therefore requires the alignment of different perspectives and the reconciliation of potentially conflicting goals (Symond *et al.* 1996).

Second, the object of work may be fragmented. It is only partially visible to participants and hence is constituted through different interests and perspectives which may be inherently contradictory. Mol (2002) has illustrated this point vividly in the healthcare context and has traced the multiple enactments through which a diagnosis of atherosclerosis is reached. She shows how the 'atherosclerosis' which is observed in the clinic differs from that brought about through the vascular laboratory, which diverges from that which is performed in the operating theatre. Mol (1999) suggests that if we accept that reality is differentially performed through a variety of practices, then there may be choices about which versions of an object is to prevail. This, she argues, requires us to consider where such options are situated and what is at stake when a decision must be taken between alternative versions (see, for example, Latimer 2000). Mol proposes that different versions of an object might interfere with each other and calls for empirical examination of how these interferences are handled in practice.

Third, the object of an activity system is always moving and because activities are mediated by artefacts, the objects of an activity must be understood within the constraints of these artefacts. Objects not only keep together the diverse elements of a given activity system, they also connect different activity systems together. Thus the object of one activity system can become a resource for (or a hindrance to) another. Thus more recent work in this field takes at least two or more interacting activity systems as the minimal unit of analysis (Engeström 2000).

My focus in this book is not with activity systems per se but with nurses' organising work. This, I argue, can be understood as arising from their positioning in relation to a number of activity systems within healthcare and the requirement to manage these inter-relationships. At one level, nurses have a central role in coordinating the diverse lines of action that contribute to the care of those patients for whom they are responsible. At another level, they have an obligation to cope with the overall work of a department, ward or caseload. Each is informed by different logics: the former is underpinned by a professional logic in which primacy is given to the needs of individuals; the latter is underpinned by a managerial logic in which primacy is given to the efficiency of the organisation in serving population needs. These two activity systems intersect and their inter-relationship must be negotiated.

In the chapters that follow, I describe nurses' organising work in terms of four domains of practice and delineate the system features from which they arise. Healthcare is knowledge intensive work, but there are tremendous challenges to knowledge sharing. In Chapter 2 I examine the nursing contribution to information flows and show how, through the development,

LIVERPOOL JOHN MOORES UNIVERSITY
LEARNING SERVICES

maintenance and circulation of 'trajectory narratives', nurses create a working knowledge to support service delivery. Chapter 3 explores the role of nurses in articulating trajectories of care. Although nurses are not typically regarded as the central actor in healthcare teams, I argue that they have a leading role in instigating, enrolling and aligning the diverse array of actors necessary to meet patient need and in ensuring that these different elements cohere. In Chapter 4 I analyse the nursing contribution to bed management. One of the most effective means of guaranteeing that patients receive the right intervention at the right time with the right outcome is by allocating beds appropriately. In the context of intensified bed utilisation in the acute sector this is ever more challenging to achieve and nurses are increasingly playing an important role here too. The final substantive chapter – Chapter 5 – explores nurses' work in facilitating the movement of patients between services. Modern healthcare organisations are highly specialised and, in a context of growing pressures to ensure that facilities are used by those who can benefit most from them, patients typically traverse multiple departments in a single episode of care. Each of the gaps between units represents potential threats to quality and safety and nurses are essential to the mitigation of these risks. Chapter 6 offers a synthesis of these findings and considers their implications. Taken together, I argue that nurses are the network builders in healthcare systems. Barely anything happens which does not pass through the hands of a nurse. As obligatory passage points, nurses are the system enablers, and their organising practices result in 'translational mobilisation', an essential but largely taken-for-granted ingredient in healthcare delivery which ensures progress and coherence where the strain towards stasis and fragmentation is ever-present.

Conclusion

This chapter has introduced the research on which this book is based. I began by developing the case for bringing about a figure-ground reversal in order to shine a light on nurses' organising work. Nurses have long been charged with this function, but it has never been the subject of serious study and has tended to be described using negative metaphors. As the literature on other kinds of invisible work has shown, this non-recognition can be highly consequential for both workers and organisations. There has been much debate about the nursing contribution to society in recent years, but this has been predicated largely on an essentialist conceptualisation of the nursing role. Taking the work of hospital nurses as the object of concern, the aim of this book is to contribute to these deliberations through the empirical analysis of the work nurses actually do and an understanding of the wider system of which they are a part. At a time of growing concern with fundamental care standards, writing about organising work runs somewhat counter to the current zeitgeist. But before we engage in debates about so-called non-nursing duties, there is a case to be made for better understanding this component of nurses' role and the circumstances that make it necessary. Only then can we reach informed decisions about delegation and substitution and only then can we consider the implications this has for nurse education, workforce planning and the quality of services. Modern healthcare systems face unparalleled pressures and there has been growing acknowledgement of the part health professionals might play in strengthening organisation and delivery. My aim here is to examine and foreground the nursing contribution to these processes.

Note

1 This extract has been fabricated for illustrative purposes.

References

Abbott, A. (1988). *The System of Professions: An Essay on the Division of Expert Labor*. Chicago, University of Chicago Press.

Aiken, L.H., Sermeus, W., Van den Heed, K., Sloane, D.M., Busse, R., McKee, M., Bruyneel, L., Rafferty, A.M., Griffiths, P., Moreno-Casbas, M.T., Tishelman, C., Scott, A., Brzostek, T., Kinnunen, J., Schwendimann, E., Heinen, M., Zikos, D., Sjetne, I.S., Smith, H.L. and A. Kutney-Lee (2012). 'Patient safety, satisfaction, and quality of hospital care: cross sectional surveys of nurses and patients in 12 countries in Europe and the United States.' *BMJ* 344(1717): 1–14.

Allen, D. (1997). 'The medical-nursing boundary: a negotiated order?' *Sociology of Health & Illness* 19(4): 498–520.

—— (2000a). '"I'll tell you what suits me best if you don't mind me saying': lay participation in health-care.' *Nursing Inquiry* 7(3): 182–190.

—— (2000b). 'Negotiating the role of expert carers on an adult hospital ward.' *Sociology of Health & Illness* 22(2): 149–171.

—— (2001a). *The Changing Shape of Nursing Practice: The Role of Nurses in the Hospital Division of Labour*. London, Routledge.

—— (2001b). 'Narrating nursing jurisdiction: atrocity stories and boundary work.' *Symbolic Interaction* 24(1): 75–103.

—— (2004). 'Re-reading nursing and re-writing practice: towards an empirically-based reformulation of the nursing mandate.' *Nursing Inquiry* 11(4): 271–283.

—— (2007). 'What did you do at work today? Profession-building and doing nursing.' *International Nursing Review* 54(1): 41–48.

—— (2009). 'From boundary concept to boundary object: the politics and practices of care pathway development.' *Social Science & Medicine* 69: 354–361.

—— (2010a). 'Care pathways: an ethnographic description of the field.' *International Journal of Care Pathways* 14: 47–51.

—— (2010b). 'Care pathways: some social scientific observations on the field.' *International Journal of Care Pathways* 14: 4–9.

Allen, D., Griffiths, L. and P. Lyne (2004). 'Understanding complex trajectories in health and social care provision.' *Sociology of Health & Illness* 26(7): 1008–1030.

Allen, D. and A. Pilnick (2005). 'Making connections: healthcare as a case study in the social organisation of work.' *Sociology of Health & Illness* 27(6): 683–700.

Annandale, E. (1996). 'Working on the front-line: risk culture and nursing in the new NHS.' *Sociological Review* 44(3): 416–451.

Armstrong, D. (1983). 'The fabrication of nurse-patient relationships.' *Social Science & Medicine* **17**(8): 457–460.

—— (1998). 'Decline of the hospital: reconstructing institutional dangers.' *Sociology of Health & Illness* **20**(4): 445–457.

Beardshaw, V. and R. Robinson (1990). *New for old? Prospects for Nursing in the 1990s*. London, King's Fund Institute.

Becker, H.S. (1970). The nature of profession. *Sociological Work*. Chicago, Aldine: 87–103.

Berg, M. (1996). 'Practices of reading and writing: the constitutive role of the patient record in medical work.' *Sociology of Health & Illness* **18**(4): 499–562.

—— (1997). 'Problems and promises of the protocol.' *Social Science & Medicine* **44**(8): 1081–1088.

—— (1997). *Rationalizing Medical Work: Decision-Support Techniques and Medical Practices*. Cambridge, Cambridge University Press.

—— (1998). Order(s) and disorder(s): of protocols and medical practices. *Differences in Medicine: Unravelling practices, techniques, and bodies*. M. Berg and A. Mol. Durham and London, Duke University Press: 226–246.

—— (1999). 'Accumulating and coordinating: occasions for information technologies in medical work.' *Computer Supported Cooperative Work* **8**: 373–401.

Bevan, H. (2010). 'How can we build skills to transform the healthcare system?' *Journal of Research in Nursing* **15**(2): 139–148.

Blum, A.F. and P. McHugh (1971). 'The social ascription of motives.' *American Sociological Review* **36**(December): 98–109.

Bolton, S. (2000). 'Who cares? Offering emotion work as a "gift" in the nursing labour process.' *Journal of Advanced Nursing* **32**(3): 580–586.

—— (2001). 'Changing faces: nurses as emotional jugglers.' *Sociology of Health & Illness* **23** (1): 85–100.

Bourdieu, P. (1977). *Outline of a Theory of Practice*. Cambridge, Cambridge University Press.

—— (1990). *The Logic of Practice*. Cambridge, Polity.

—— (2000). *Pascalian Meditations*. Stanford, CA, Stanford University Press.

Bowker, G.C., Starr, S.L. and M.A. Spasser (2001). 'Classifying nursing work.' *Online Journal of Issues in Nursing* **6**(2). www.nursingworld.org/MainMenu Categories/ANAMarketplace/ANAPeriodicals/OJIN/TableofContents/Volume 62001/No2May01/ArticlePreviousTopic/ClassifyingNursingWork.aspx (accessed 3 May 2013).

Brown, S.D. (2002). 'Michel Serres: science, translation and the logic of the parasite.' *Theory, Culture and Society* **19**(3): 1–27.

Callon, M. (1986). Some elements of a sociology of translation: domestication of the scallops and the fishermen of St Brieuc Bay. *Power, Action and Belief: A New Sociology of Knowledge*. J. Law. London, Routledge & Kegan Paul: 196–229.

—— (1991). Techno-economic networks and irreversibility. *A Sociology of Monsters: Essays on Power, Technology and Domination*. J. Law. London, Routledge: 132–161.

Carpenter, M. (1977). The new managerialism and professionalism in nursing. *Health and the Division of Labour*. M. Stacey, M. Reid, C. Heath and R. Dingwall. London, Croom Helm: 120–42.

Charles-Jones, H., Latimer, J. and C. May (2003). 'Transforming General Practice: the redistribution of medical work in primary care.' *Sociology of Health & Illness* **25**(1): 71–92.

Cohen, R.L. (2011). 'Time, space and touch at work: body work and labour process (re)organisation.' *Sociology of Health & Illness* 33(2): 189–205.

Crawford, C.S. (2004). Actor network theory. *Encyclopedia of Social Theory*. G. Ritzer. Thousand Oaks, California, Sage.

Crawford, P. and B. Brown (2008). 'Soft authority: ecologies of infection management in the working lives of modern matrons and infection control staff.' *Sociology of Health & Illness* 30(5): 756–771.

Cressman, D. (2009). *A Brief Overview of Actor-network Theory: Punctualization, Hetergeneous Engineering & Translation*, ACT Lab/Centre for Policy Research on Science & Technology, School Of Communication, Simon Fraser University.

Davies, C. (1995). *Gender and the Professional Predicament in Nursing*. Buckingham, Open University Press.

Davies, C. (2012). 'London hospital blamed for man's dehydration death.' www. guardian.co.uk/society/2012/jul/12/london-hospital-kane-gorny-dehydration-death (accessed 14 July 2012).

Dear, M. and S. Flusty (2002). *The Spaces of Postmodernity: Readings in Human Geography*. Oxford, Blackwell Publishers.

Dent, M. (1999). 'Professional judgement and the role of clinical guidelines and evidence-based medicine (EBM): Netherlands, Britain and Sweden.' *Journal of Interprofessional Care* 13(2): 151–164.

DiMaggio, P.J. and W.W. Powell (1983). 'The iron cage revisited: institutional isomorphism and collective rationality in organizational fields.' *American Sociological Review* 48(April): 147–160.

Dingwall, R. (1983). 'In the begining was the work... reflections on the genesis of occupations.' *Sociological Review* 31: 605–624.

Dingwall, R. and D. Allen (2001). 'The implications of healthcare reforms for the profession of nursing.' *Nursing Inquiry* 8(2): 64–74.

Durkheim, E. (1933). *The Division of Labour in Society*. London, Collier-Macmillan Ltd.

Engeström, Y. (2000). 'Activity Theory as a framework for analysing and redesigning work.' *Ergonomics* 43(7): 960–972.

—— (2008). *From Teams to Knots: Activity Theoretical Studies of Collaboration and Learning at Work*. Cambridge, Cambridge University Press.

Engeström, Y., Engeström, R. and T. Vähääho (2002). When the centre does not hold: the importance of knotworking. *Activity Theory and Social Practice: Cultural-Historical approaches*. S. Chaiklin, H. Hedegaard and U.J. Jensen: 345–374.

Freidland, R. and R.R. Alford (1991). Bringing society back in: symbols, practices and institutional contradictions. *The New Institutionalism in Organizational Analysis*. W.W. Powell and P.J. DiMaggio. Chicago, University of Chicago Press: 232–263.

Freidson, E. (1976). 'The division of labour as social interaction.' *Social Problems* 23: 304–313.

Furaker, C. (2009). 'Nurses' everyday activities in hospital care.' *Journal of Nursing Management* 17(3): 269–277.

Gabriel, Y. (1993). Organizational nostalgia – reflections on the 'golden age'. *Emotion in Organization*. S. Fineman. London, Sage: 118–141.

Garfinkel, H. (1967). *Studies in Ethnomethodology*. New Jersey, Prentice Hall.

Gerth, H. and C.W. Mills (1946). *From Max Weber: Essay in Sociology*. New York, Oxford University Press.

Gherardi, S. and D. Nicolini (2005). Actor networks: ecology and entrepeneurs. *Actor-Network Theory and Organizing.* B. Czarniawska and T. Hernes. Malmo, Sweden, Liber and Copenhagen Business School Press: 285–306.

Giddens, A. (1984). *The Constitution of Society: Outline of a Theory of Structuration.* Cambridge, Polity Press.

Glen, S. (2004). 'Healthcare reforms: implications for the education and training of acute and critical care nurses.' *Postgraduate Medical Journal* 80: 706–710.

Hampson, I. and A. Junor (2005). 'Invisible work, invisible skills: interactive customer service as articulation work.' *New Technology, Work and Employment* 20(2): 166–181.

—— (2010). 'Putting the process back in: rethinking service sector skill.' *Work, Employment and Society* 24(3): 526–545.

Hart, L. (1991). A ward of my own: social organisation and identity among hospital domestics. *Anthropology and Nursing.* P. Holden and J. Littleworth. London, Routledge: 84–109.

Henderson, V. (1966). *The Nature of Nursing.* New York, Macmillan Publishing.

Horton, R. (1997). Health: a complicated game of doctors and nurses. *Observer.* London.

House of Commons (2010). Independent Inquiry into Care Provided by Mid Staffordshire NHS Foundation Trust January 2005 – March 2009, Volumes I and II, (Chaired by Robert Francis QC), HC375. London, The Stationery Office.

—— (2013). Report of the Mid Staffordshire NHS Foundation Trust Public Inquiry, Volumes I, II and III (Chaired by Robert Francis QC), HC 898. London, The Stationery Office.

Hughes, E.C. (1951). 'Studying the nurses' work.' *The American Journal of Nursing* 51: 294–295.

—— (1984). *The Sociological Eye.* New Brunswick & London, Transaction Books.

Hughes, E.C., Hughes, H. and I. Deutscher (1958). *Twenty Thousand Nurses Tell Their Story.* Philadelphia, JB Lippincott.

Hutchby, I. (2001). 'Technology, texts and affordances.' *Sociology* 35: 411–456.

James, N. (1989). 'Emotional labour: skill and work in the social regulation of feelings.' *Sociological Review* 37(1): 15–42.

—— (1992). 'Care = organisation + physical labour = emotional labour.' *Sociology of Health & Illness* 14(4): 488–509.

Kitchener, M. (2002). 'Mobilising the logic of managerialism in professional fields: the case of Academic Health Centers mergers.' *Organization Studies* 23(3): 391–420.

Latimer, J. (2000). *The Conduct of Care: Understanding Nursing Practice.* Oxford, Blackwells.

Latour, B. (1991). Technology is society made durable. *A Sociology of Monsters: Essays on Power, Technology and Domination.* J. Law. London, Routledge: 103–131.

—— (1998). Mixing humans and nonhumans together: the sociology of a door-closer. *Ecologies of Knowledge: Work and Politics in Science and Technology.* S.L. Star. New York, State University of New York Press: 257–277.

—— (2005). *Reassembling the Social: An Introduction to Actor-Network-Theory.* Oxford, Oxford University Press.

Law, J. (1992). 'Notes on the theory of the actor-network: ordering, strategy and heterogeneity.' *Systems Practice* 5: 379–393.

Law, J. and M. Callon (1988). 'Engineering and sociology in a military aircraft project: a network analysis of technological change.' *Social Problems* 35(3): 284–297.

—— (1994). The life or death of an aircraft: a network analysis of technical change. *Shaping Technology/Building Society: Studies in Sociotechnical Change*. W.E. Bijker and J. Law. Cambridge, Massachusetts, MIT Press: 21–52.

Law, J. and J. Hassard, Eds. (1999). *Actor Network Theory and After*. Oxford, Blackwell Publishing.

Lawler, J. (1991). *Behind the Screens: Nursing, Somology and the Problem of the Body*. London, Churchill Livingstone.

Lawson, N. (1996). Is this the end nurses? *The Times*. London.

Maben, J. and P. Griffiths (2008). Nurses in Society: Starting the Debate. London, National Nursing Research Unit: King's College London, University of London.

Maben, J., Latter, S. and J. Macleod-Clark (2006). 'The theory-practice gap: the impact of professional-bureaucratic work conflict on the experiences of newly qualified nurses in the UK.' *Journal of Advanced Nursing* 55(4): 465–477.

Mauksch, H.O. (1966). Organisational context of nursing practice. *The Nursing Profession*. F. Davis. New York, Wiley: 109–137.

May, C. (1992). 'Nursing work, nurses' knowledge, and the subjectification of the patient.' *Sociology of Health & Illness* 14(4): 472–487.

McDonald, R. and S. Harrison (2004). 'The micropolitics of clinical guidelines: an empirical study.' *Policy & Politics* 32 (2): 223–239.

Messman, J. (2008). *Uncertainty in Medical Innovation: Experienced Pioneers in Neonatal Care*. Basingstoke, Palgrave Macmillan.

Meyer, J.W. and B. Rowan (1977). 'Institutionalized organizations: formal structure as myth and ceremony.' *American Journal of Sociology* 83(2): 340–363.

Mills, C.W. (1940). 'Situated actions and vocabularies of motive.' *American Sociological Review* 5 (February): 904–913.

Mol, A. (1999). Ontological politics: A word and some questions. *Actor Network Theory and After*. J. Law and J. Hassard. Oxford, Blackwell Publishing: 74–89.

—— (2002). *The Body Multiple: Ontology in Medical Practice*. Durham, NC, Duke University Press.

Morrow, E., Robert, G., Maben, J. and P. Griffiths (2012). 'Implementing large-scale quality improvement: lessons from The Productive Ward: Releasing Time to Care™.' *International Journal of Health Care Quality Assurance* 25(4): 237–253.

Mort, M., May, C., Finch, T. and F. Mair (2004). Telemedicine and clinical governance: controlling technology, controlling knowledge. *Governing Medicine: Theory and Practice*. A. Gray and S. Harrison. Berkshire, OUP: 107–121.

Muller, M.J. (1999). 'Invisible work of telephone operators: an ethnocritical analysis.' *Computer Support Cooperative Work* 8: 31–61.

Nardi, B. and R. Engeström (1999). 'A web on the wind: the structure of invisible work.' *Computer Support Cooperative Work* 8: 1–8.

Nelson, S. and S. Gordon (2006). *The Complexities of Care: Nursing Reconsidered*. Ithaca, ILR Press.

Nicolini, D. (2012). *Practice Theory, Work and Organization: An Introduction*. Oxford, Oxford University Press.

Nightingale, F. (1860/1969). *Notes on Nursing and Other Writings*. New York, Dover Publications Inc.

Ortner, S. (1984). 'Theory in anthropology since the sixties.' *Comparative Studies in Society and History* 26(1): 126–166.

Osborne, S., Radnor, Z.J. and G. Nasi (2012). 'A new theory for public service management? Towards a service-dominant approach.' *American Review of Public Administration* arp.sagepub.com/content/early/2012/12/04/0275074012466935

Paterson, E. (1981). Food-work: maids in a hospital kitchen. *Medical Work*. P. Atkinson and C. Heath. Farnborough, Gower: 152–170.

Pols, J. (2010a) 'Caring devices. About warmth, coldness and care that fits.' *Medische Antropologie* **22**(1): 143–160.

—— (2010b) 'The heart of the matter. About good nursing and telecare.' *Health Care Analysis* **18**(4): 374–388.

—— (2012). *Care at a Distance: On the Closeness of Technology*. Amsterdam, Amsterdam University Press.

Pols, J. and D. Willems (2011). 'Innovation and evaluation. Taming and unleashing telecare technologies.' *Sociology of Health & Illness* **33**(4): 484–498.

Power, M. (1997). *The Audit Society: Rituals of Verification*. Oxford, Oxford University Press.

Purkis, M.E. (2001). 'Managing home care: visibility, accountability and exclusion.' *Nursing Inquiry* **8**: 141–150.

Purkis, M.E. and K. Bjornsdottir (2006). 'Intelligent nursing: accounting for knowledge as action in practice.' *Nursing Philosophy* **7**: 247–256.

Quested, B. and T. Rudge (2002). 'Nursing care of dead bodies: a discursive analysis of last offices.' *Journal of Advanced Nursing* **41**(6): 553–560.

Radnor, Z.J. and S.P. Osborne (2013). 'Lean: a failed theory for public management.' *Public Management Review* **15**(2): 265–287.

Rollins, J. (1985). *Between Women*. Boston, Beacon Press.

Royal College of Nursing (2003). 'Defining Nursing.' www.rcn.org.uk/__data/assets/pdf_file/0008/78569/001998.pdf (accessed 13 June 2013).

Rudge, T. (2009). 'Beyond caring? Discounting the differently known body.' *Sociological Review* **56**(s2): 233–248.

Ruef, M. and W.R. Scott (1998). 'A multidimensional model of organizational legitimacy: hospital survival in changing institutional environments.' *Administrative Science Quarterly* **43**(4): 877–904.

Sandelowski, M. (2000). *Devices & Desires: Gender, Technology, and American Nursing*. Chapel Hill, North Carolina Press.

Scott, C. and S.M. Lyman (1968). 'Accounts.' *American Sociological Review* **22**(Feburary): 46–62.

Scott, W.R. (1977). Effectiveness of organizational effectiveness studies. *New perspectives on Organizational Effectiveness*. P.S. Goodman and J.M. Pennings. San Francisco, Jossey-Bass: 63–95.

—— (2004). Competing logics in health care: professional, state, and managerial. *The Sociology of the Economy*. F. Dobbin. New York, Russell Sage Foundation: 276–287.

—— (2005). Institutional theory: contributing to a theoretical research program. *Great Minds in Management: The Process of Theory Development*. K.G. Smith and M.A. Hitt. Oxford, Oxford University Press: 460–484.

Scott, W.R. and J.W. Meyer (1983). The organization of societal sectors. *Organizational Environments: Ritual and rationality*. J.W. Meyer and W.R. Scott. Beverly Hills, CA, Sage: 129–153.

Selznick, P. (1957). *Leadership in Administration*. New York, Harper & Row.

Smith, P. (1992). *The Emotional Labour of Nursing*. London, Macmillan.

Smith, P. and B. Gray (2001). 'Reassessing the concept of emotional labour in student nurse education: role of link lecturers and mentors in a time of change.' *Nurse Education Today* 21: 230–237.

Spradley, J.P. (1980). *Participant Observation*. Orlando, Florida, Holt, Rinehart and Winston, Inc.

Star, S.L. and A. Strauss (1999). 'Layers of silence, arenas of voice: the ecology of visible and invisible work.' *Computer Supported Cooperative Work* 8: 9–30.

Strauss, A., Fagerhaugh, S. and B. Suczet (1985). *The Social Organization of Medical Work*. Chicago, University of Chicago Press.

Stroebaek, P.S. (2013). 'Lets have a cup of coffee! Coffee and coping communities at work.' *Symbolic Interaction* 36(4): 381–397.

Suchman, L. (1995). 'Making work visible.' *Communications of the ACM* 38(9): 56–64.

—— (1987). *Plans and Situated Actions. The Problem of Human-Machine Communication*. Cambridge, Cambridge University Press.

Suchman, M.C. (1995). 'Managing legitimacy: strategic and institutional approaches.' *Academy of Management Review* 20(3): 571–610.

Symond, G., Long, K. and J. Ellis (1996). 'The coordination of work activities: cooperation and conflict in a hospital context.' *Computer Supported Cooperative Work: The Journal of Collaborative Computing* 5: 1–31.

Theodosius, C. (2008). *Emotional Labour in Health Care: The Unmanaged Heart of Nursing*. London and New York, Routledge.

Thorton, P.H. and W. Ocasio (2008). Institutional logics. *The Sage Handbook of Organizational Institutionalism*. R. Greenwood, C. Oliver, R. Suddaby and K. Sahlin-Andersson. London, Sage: 99–129.

Tjora, A. (2000). 'The technological mediation of the nursing-medical boundary.' *Sociology of Health & Illness* 22: 721–741.

Traynor, M. (2009). 'Indeterminacy and technicality revisited: how medicine and nursing have responded to the evidence based movement.' *Sociology of Health & Illness* 31(4): 494–507.

Twigg, J., Wolkowitz, C., Cohen, R.L. and S. Nettleton (2011). 'Conceptualising body work in health and social care.' *Sociology of Health & Illness* 33(2): 171–188.

UKCC (1987). *Project 2000: The Final Proposals*. London, UKCC.

Weick, K.E. (1995). *Sensemaking in Organizations*. Thousand Oaks, London, New Dehli, Sage.

Westerberg, K. (1999). 'Collaborative networks among female middle managers in a hierarchical organization.' *Computer Supported Cooperative Work* 8: 95–114.

Whittaker, E.W. and V.L. Olesen (1964). 'The faces of Florence Nightingale: functions of the heroine legend in an occupational culture.' *Human Organization* 23: 123–130.

2 Creating working knowledge

There is, quite literally, no single individual who possesses the complete knowledge about any given patient.

(Ellingsen and Monteiro 2003: 204)

Healthcare is knowledge-intensive work. Whether it is for treatment, rehabilitation or palliation, meeting patients' needs is an intellectually intricate activity involving numerous individuals with discrete expertise. Not surprisingly, then, knowledge management is a central preoccupation of hospital organisation with significant resources committed to accumulating, documenting and sharing information. Despite such investment, for the purposes of ongoing patient care much of the day-to-day work of knowledge generation is undertaken by nurses and while it may be true that no single individual possesses complete understanding of specific patients, nurses come closest to holding this global view. In this chapter I examine the work nurses do to create the knowledge flows which support the practical delivery of healthcare. In a dynamic environment in which the needs of patients and the shape of the organisation change rapidly this is a significant undertaking.

The challenges of knowledge-sharing

We are very fond of using the language of 'team' to describe healthcare work, but to a considerable extent patient care is progressed through *individual* rather than collaborative activity. In a world of super specialisation, multiple actors make largely independent contributions to individual cases and their work is widely distributed across time and space. Each operates with a different and partial version of the patient, reflecting their singular work purposes, distinctive professional gaze (Foucault 1973; Armstrong 1983; May 1992; Barber 2005) and the tools with which they practise (Mol 2002). Thus, for much of the time, facts and understanding pertinent to an individual's care are dispersed throughout a diverse network of health professionals, communities, artefacts and information systems (Ellingsen and Monteiro 2003). Although it is not uncommon for participants in collaborative work situations to vary in the knowledge they possess, arrangements must be in place to enable them to pool resources and negotiate to accomplish their tasks.[1] The greater the heterogeneity and complexity of knowledge sources in an activity system and the more understanding has to be achieved across time and space, the bigger is the challenge of achieving this (Bossen 2002). The demands of knowledge-sharing that confront healthcare organisations are compounded by the emergent and contingent nature of the work. Trajectories of care, as I have argued, are unpredictable and their management is intricately bound up with the changing shape of the organisation and such vicissitudes must be responded to. Yet despite the complex, fragmented and emergent nature of healthcare delivery, it is only rarely, if ever, that *all* participants come together to share information and align their work activities. Formal coordinating events such as team meetings and ward rounds are important mechanisms for knowledge mobilisation, but compared to the speed with which trajectories evolve these are relatively infrequent events.

The patient record is widely recognised as the central medium of inter-professional communication in healthcare and in recent years, as service integration has become progressively more important, there has been substantial investment in new information systems to support knowledge-sharing, albeit with mixed results (Greenhalgh *et al.* 2009). Historically an educational tool, consisting of loosely structured descriptions of particular cases in a narrative format (Seigler 2010), the patient record has since evolved to become a highly complex account of any aspect of treatment which has official status within a healthcare system (Berg and Bowker 1997). At one level, an ever-more specialised division of labour and the aspiration for integrated care has increased its complexity, such that what was once exclusively a medical record is now a multidisciplinary tool. At another level, in a context in which trust in health professionals has been replaced by trust in auditable systems (Power 1997), formal documentation has become important evidence of organisational and professional performance and a mechanism by which legitimacy can be secured. This has precipitated a shift towards the detailed citation of specific accountable interventions, in highly structured and codified formats that can be readily audited and, as a result, the contemporary patient record is an intricate combination of free-text entries, checklists, reports, charts, care plans, pathways, risk assessments and other proforma. Far from serving as a straightforward presentation of clinical data, it embodies multiple, fragmented representations of the patient (Berg and Bowker 1997; Mol 2002) created for diverse clinical and organisational purposes. While these may function to demonstrate that the organisation is making proper efforts to ensure the quality of its processes, for the purposes of ongoing service delivery, synthesising patient information from such a complex assemblage is a demanding task.

Whether paper-based or electronic, the formal record may be conceptualised either as an 'information repository' or as a 'record at work in the practical delivery of healthcare' (Fitzpatrick 2004). Another way of expressing these differences is to distinguish between the 'archival patient record' and the 'working patient record' (Fitzpatrick 2004). Healthcare organisations are underpinned by the assumption that the medical record is able to serve both purposes and a number of recent information technologies have been promulgated on this basis. Thus, the shift from mono-professional to multi-professional records was driven in part by the aspiration to support care coordination and create unified documentation. Similarly, integrated care pathways have been promoted as both a workflow model and a mechanism for accounting for practice (Allen 2009, 2010a, b). A good example of how dominant management logics are increasingly penetrating the technical aspects of healthcare work, this dual functionality is not without its tensions, and the growing demand for greater transparency and performance management has increasingly emphasised those features of the medical record which support its archival purposes, but as a consequence rendered it less able to operate as a working patient record. Many of the disappointments relating to the utility of new electronic record systems are that these have been designed for data collection, rather than for use by healthcare workers in daily clinical practice (Coiera 1997). Thus, while the formal record may support individual lines of action and discrete interventions, for the purposes of the ongoing coordination of an overall trajectory of care it is insufficient. Indeed, nowhere in the formal record does a documented summative version of the current status of the patient's trajectory exist.

This is not to say that formal records do not matter; they do. Action must be documented in the appropriate place; it is a professional and organisational requirement. But while these materials contribute in fundamental ways to the ordering of healthcare and how trajectories are understood, represented, made sense of and accounted for, empirical examination of real-life healthcare work reveals that on their own they have limited value for the purposes of everyday work organisation. Trajectories and organisations move too quickly and the daily pressures of the acute hospital, where multiple trajectories are managed simultaneously, require a more agile approach. It is nurses who fulfil this function. Nurses at Parklands expended considerable energy in locating, validating, double-checking and interpreting relevant information sources, which they then translated into narratives that stabilised and gave sense to individual trajectories of care. It was through this largely invisible work that nurses functioned to create working knowledge (Ellingsen and Monteiro 2003) for the purposes of organising ongoing activity.

A central resource

'Well we're the link really, the dieticians and the physios and everyone tell us and then we communicate it to everyone else.'

'They ((doctors)) spend so little time on the ward it's up to us to fill them in.'

The main components of the coordinator role are: 'Knowing exactly what's going on everywhere.'

In the hospital setting, nurses work continuously in the sites of care whereas other providers operate across a wider landscape and offer temporally intermittent services. In the daily comings and goings of health professionals and service managers around patients, nurses function as an important central information source and a common link. Personnel attending the clinical areas on an itinerant basis might well consult formal technologies to seek out information, but it was normal practice to enter into discussion with nursing staff too.

A doctor comes onto the ward and studies the white board.

Doctor: 'Any issues?'

Ward Manager: 'With whom?'

Doctor: 'Monday team patients?'

Coordinator: 'We need a medical review of this one ((points to white board)) no this one' ((points to another bed space)).

As we will see in Chapter 3, nurses have a central role in coordinating the ongoing organisation of healthcare delivery and in order to undertake this function they must generate and keep in play a working knowledge of the evolving status of patient trajectories. This requires oversight individual's unfolding needs the changing shape of the organisation and the intersection of these two systems. In some areas, responsibility for both functions was assumed by the ward coordinator who acted as a single point of contact and interceded between the nurses caring for patients clinically, the wider network of healthcare providers and service managers. In other areas, the professed purpose of the coordinator was to manage the ward or unit and to expedite discharge processes, but responsibility for individual trajectory management resided with the nurses providing direct patient care. Neither of these arrangements was without its tensions, however, and in practice the separation of roles as described here was fuzzier than these distinctions imply, with nurses working organically and flexibly in response to contingencies as they arose. Indeed, for reasons I will elaborate upon later, there was a view that nurses worked most successfully in creating a working knowledge when they operated as a single actor.

Central to nurses' knowledge mobilisation work was the trajectory narrative. Trajectory narratives are narratives of encapsulation (Knorr-Cetina 1999) which function to sustain a working record of individuals' ongoing care. They were created by nurses when a patient was admitted to the service and thereafter set into circulation through the nursing handover. Nurses recorded the salient details of trajectory narratives on sheets of paper. These 'plot summaries' functioned as an aide memoire for the purposes of ongoing work organisation and could readily be updated. This is important, because narratives did not remain static. Nurses revised their content over the course of their everyday work, through scrutiny of the medical record, attendance at ward rounds and team meetings and in dialogue with the network of actors involved in a given patient's care. Narratives were modified in their numerous tellings too, with nurses adjusting their content to meet the needs of different audiences and the circumstances at hand.

Creating trajectory narratives

When a patient was admitted to a service, nurses undertook initial work to establish the events that had precipitated their need for healthcare. Doctors and other healthcare providers assembled their own histories too, the content reflecting their particular work purposes. The nursing admission process was distinctive, however, insofar as it extended beyond nursing interventions and entailed work to assemble a wider picture of the patient, their overall health and social care needs, and the story of this admission. Indeed, the notion of a 'nursing assessment' is somewhat misleading; nurses oriented to the whole trajectory in their information-seeking.

On a daily basis, nursing handover was the central mechanism through which trajectory narratives were set into circulation. As with the admission process, however, the term 'nursing handover' is an inexact descriptor of what actually occurs on such occasions. First, the work that is accomplished is more complex than a simple transfer of information. For each patient, nurses told the story of their evolving trajectory of care. Typically presented chronologically, narratives were not only an account of what had occurred over the previous shift as the term handover implies, they also looked back to what had taken place in the past (perhaps even before the patient was admitted to hospital) and forward to planned activity. Some of this information would be available in the official record, but not in the same form. Rather, the trajectory narrative was a synthesis based on reading the notes, previous handovers, interpretative understanding and experience of the case, as well as an assessment of the immediate requirements of the situation and the information needs of the receiving nurse. The organisation and content of handovers was variable in different settings, but their form was remarkably consistent.[2] Second, to call such occasions a *nursing* handover is also deceptive. While incorporating details on nursing interventions, trajectory narratives included information about the contribution of others too. Indeed, they encapsulated a global view of individuals' overall care, integrating clinical information about patients' progress with the contextual and organisational information necessary for coordinating work activity. This is why, building on Strauss *et al.* (1985), I have called them *trajectory* narratives (see Chapter 1).

Within the nursing body, the construction of trajectory narratives was a collaborative activity. Nurses worked together during handover to assemble a picture of the patient, their care and the associated resources and activity. The following extract is a typical example. The night nurse is handing over to the coordinator who had been working the previous day. The extract begins with the night nurse explaining that the patient is a new admission, indicating that her trajectory is short and uncertain. On several occasions the nurse identifies areas of incomplete knowledge and the coordinator responds by filling in information fragments where she can. What emerges is a clearer picture of the patient in which some gaps in understanding are resolved, and issues requiring clarification identified.

> Night Staff Nurse: 'Bed 3 [...] a new lady, 84, came in with a fall and broken arm. She has a POP ((plaster cast)) in situ. She's on 12 hourly obs and is to be seen in Fracture Clinic in a week. She's for a 24-hour tape to see whether her fall was due to arrhythmias. She's mobile over short distances but has some shortness of breath. She's been using a commode over night. I don't know what she's like during the day.'

> Coordinator: 'I didn't have chance to assess her with all that was going on yesterday.'

> Night Staff Nurse: 'She is a smoker and we need the doctor to assess whether she wants a nicotine patch or anything. She lives alone but I am not sure how well she copes.'

> Coordinator: 'Her daughter spoke to me yesterday and said that she is no longer coping at home so we need to make a social worker referral.'

Trajectory narratives are dynamic artefacts. They were revised and renewed by nurses as part of their ongoing work activity during which they accumulated, made sense of and synthesised information from a number of sources. While of limited direct value for the purposes of everyday care coordination, nurses used the medical record in order to elaborate upon and fill in any gaps in their understanding. A number of respondents volunteered that they liked to consult the medical record to supplement the information given at handover. Reviewing the medical notes was considered to be particularly important if the nurse had returned from days off or where the handover had indicated some uncertainty about the current status of a trajectory.

Formal coordination events were also significant for the maintenance of trajectory narratives. The ward round, the frequency of which varied across the different units in the organisation, was essentially a medical occasion, but nurses attended if they were able. Observers of clinical practice have often noted nurses' relative passivity on the ward round, claiming that they do not appear to contribute to decision-making (Latimer 2000; Manias and Street 2001) but they are doing other important invisible work. Many of the decisions made in such fora were consequential for understanding the evolving trajectory of care, and nurses attended in order to be able to extract the information necessary to update the associated narratives.

Beyond these formal mechanisms, much of the work of maintaining the currency of trajectory narratives was accomplished through ongoing dialogue with health providers and woven through the warp and weft of everyday practice. As I have argued, the knowledge pertinent to a given patient is differentially distributed between actors and while nurses were the only healthcare providers to take responsibility for knowledge creation related to overall trajectory management, others had more detailed understanding of different elements of this process. As a result of their ongoing interactions with the actors passing through the care setting nurses were made aware of new information and incorporated this into their evolving understanding of the trajectory, which they then passed on to others. The social organisation of healthcare is regularly punctuated with such moments.

> Coordinator: 'Mr [...] in the cubicle was admitted yesterday but he doesn't have a drug chart. He's taking his own meds at the moment, but he's a bit constipated and I'd like to get that sorted out before theatre.'
>
> Junior Doctor 1: 'When's he going?'
>
> Coordinator: 'Possibly Tuesday and he's possibly for a cardiac angio today.'
>
> Both junior doctors look surprised: 'Oh!'
>
> Coordinator: 'Mr [...] happened to mention it when he popped in Saturday!'

Plot summaries

Trajectory narratives are also written phenomena. Nurses in receipt of handover made a paper-based record of relevant details for their own work purposes. I intentionally positioned myself alongside the coordinators at handover so as to observe the content of these entries to gain insight into their work priorities and organising practices. At first I thought they were simply lists of jobs to do (referrals to make, documentation to be completed, medications to be prescribed) and this was of interest in understanding the content of their work. However, I also observed that their notes included details of completed actions and not just those for which nurses were responsible, but the work of others too. In the extracts below, which are reproduced from a coordinator's handover notes, we can see a number of ticked boxes indicating that the unified assessment (UA) forms 3–11 (important in managing discharge from hospital) have been completed, a social worker (SW) referral made and a hoist ordered. In the first extract there is a query about whether a patient is eligible for continuing health care (CHC) funding, in the second, the nurse documents that a case conference will be required before discharge as the patient lives alone and in the third, it is noted that the patient is to go home on Monday at 10am and that they will require blister packs (b/packs).[3]

'Drain, UA 3-11 ☑? CHC, SW'

'C/conf lives alone, SW ☑'

'Home mon 10am, b/packs, hoist ☑'

In effect, the written record of handover was a 'plot summary' of individual trajectory narratives. Whether inscribed on scraps of paper, pre-printed handover sheets, or the unit coordinator's book designated for this purpose, the handover record was a highly portable, easily accessible summation of the status of a care trajectory that could be updated instantly. It represented a synthesis and translation of information aggregated from diverse sources, in addition to intelligence that would not be found in any formal record, but which was necessary for managing the work. As such it functioned as a pragmatic condensation and encapsulation of the current status of the trajectory that was unavailable anywhere else and functioned as an important aide memoire.

> Coordinator is about to start the paperwork for the new admission when the agency nurse arrives. She is greeted very warmly indeed! Coordinator now has to hand over to the agency nurse. It is 13:30 and only half an hour since she received handover from her colleague. She then spends a further 10 minutes telling the agency nurse about patients she has had nothing to do with on the basis of the handover she received a few minutes earlier. What was remarkable about this was the similarity in the content of both handovers and how, from the few notes she had made on her sheet, she could recall the detail and context of her colleague's handover to her.

Nurses routinely conducted the inter-shift handover and contributed to multidisciplinary meetings and ward rounds from their plot summaries, not the medical or official nursing record. I also observed nurses using their handover notes as the basis for completing other documentation, such as preoperative checklists. Specialists visiting the ward, such as the stroke coordinator, borrowed them too, to identify any potential patients for referral. Indeed, the importance of nurses' handover records for the everyday organisation of nursing work is illustrated by the panic engendered when individuals thought these were lost.

> We go to the next patient who is sleeping. Coordinator thinks she is 'nil by mouth' and looks to consult his handover sheet. He can't find it.

> Coordinator: 'Don't say I've lost that already! That would be a disaster!'

Coordinator: 'Have you seen my handover sheet? I've lost it.'

Deputy Sister: 'It's like losing your memory!'

Hardey *et al.* (2000: 209) analyse nurses' use of 'scraps', which they define as the 'personalized recordings of information that is routinely made on any available piece of paper (hence scraps) or in small notebooks'. They examine the processes through which these are constructed, their use in daily practice and consider issues relating to the confidentiality of their content. They argue that scraps represent a unique combination of personal and professional knowledge that informs the delivery of care and propose that scrutiny of their substance has the potential to yield insights into nursing knowledge. I agree with this observation. The overall thrust of their argument, however, suggests that they anticipate that such an analysis will uncover nurses' unique understanding of the *care* of individual patients, in contradistinction to the biomedical focus of the medical model. My analysis points to knowledge of a different kind: nurses' working knowledge of the whole patient trajectory. There are certain clues in Hardey *et al.*'s observation that 'nurses were observed to be using scraps when providing other health and social care professionals, as well as relatives with information' (2000: 212) which points to a similar interpretation, but they do not make this extrapolation and say nothing about the content of the information contained therein. That nurses and other providers operate with working notes is well-recognised. These are essentially summaries of patient situations and designed to support information-sharing among team members (Chen 2010). Working notes are typically discarded after they have served their purpose, however, and whereas the respective interventions of other health professionals that are supported by their working notes will eventually be recorded in the formal patient record, the organising work that trajectory narratives sustain will not, a factor which contributes to its invisibility.

Sensemaking and sensegiving

The creation of working knowledge for the purposes of coordinating healthcare practice involves more than accumulating and circulating information. Decisions have to be made about what to take note of and what to ignore and the relationship between different information sources must be adjudicated. This entails sensemaking (Weick 1995). Sensemaking refers to the processes through which organisational actors try to create order when a situation does not make sense from a particular perspective. It is about meaning generation and understanding. Albolino *et al.* (2007) studied an intensive care unit and distinguished between two kinds of sensemaking: 'sensemaking-at-intervals' and 'sensemaking-on-the-fly'. Sensemaking-at-intervals referred to sensemaking during rounds and formal occasions set aside for this purpose, whereas sensemaking-on-the-fly was embedded in the ongoing work processes, for which time is not formally set aside. Much of nurses' sensemaking related to this latter kind of activity and took place under the radar of the formal organisational structure.

At Parklands, while nurses expended considerable effort accumulating information from a range of sources, there was much work involved too in validating and double-checking these and filling in gaps in understanding. Sensemaking, as Weick (1995) observes, may be triggered by a surprise, uncertainty or ambiguity. Record entries are not always clear, or a story does not hang together, creates unease or provides an insufficient basis for action. In such circumstances, nurses were observed to cross-check different sources. Thus in the following example, the night staff nurse reads from the nursing notes that a medical review is required, but it is not clear who the relevant team is and the coordinator undertakes to consult the medical notes to clarify the situation.

> Night Staff Nurse: 'She needs a review by the Orthopods.'
>
> Coordinator: 'Who's she under? She's not been seen by anyone?'
>
> Night Staff Nurse: 'It says to be seen on the ward round today.'
>
> Coordinator: 'We'll see which team she's under. I'll check in the notes.'

As we will see in Chapter 5, patients typically traverse multiple interfaces in a typical episode of care and this often entails transferring information from one set of documents to another. In the course of this process, information can, and did, get lost or was inaccurately recorded. Extra time was required to clarify the 'facts' and construct a narrative that made sense given what was known about the clinical details of the case, and the operation of the organisation, its routines and patterns of activity.

> Coordinator: 'He has two black eyes which he didn't have before theatre.'
>
> Staff Nurse: 'I spoke to the recovery nurse and it's not from taping his eyes as it's in the wrong place. It looks like where they pushed the ((anaesthetic)) mask down too hard.'

Research on medical decision-making has shown that when actors make sense of information they assess the credibility of the source and this is tightly linked to the status of the responsible individual (Cicourel 1990). My data shows another set of considerations in play, nurses' knowledge work also depended on their understanding of clinical patterns and organisational routines.

> Night Staff Nurse: 'In cubicle [...] 75, subtotal gastrectomy. He's an ERAS ((Enhanced Recovery After Surgery Pathway)) patient. He's got E. coli in his wound.'
>
> Staff Nurse: 'That's a funny place to get E. coli.'

Night Staff Nurse: 'Bed 3 [...] 74 year old lady. I can't understand this transfer as she came from Gynae but she was under urology. I didn't think you could transfer from an outlier to an outlier.'

Staff Nurse: 'You can't; not really.'

Trajectories out of alignment with organisationally recognisable formats attracted attention and prompted sensemaking. As I will argue in the next chapter, patterns, routines and standards are central to the organisation of healthcare work, although perhaps not in the ways commonly assumed. They are both triggers for sensemaking and the *resources* through which it can proceed.

Sensemaking is often confused with interpretation, but there are important differences. Whereas interpretation is about understanding, sensemaking also includes enactment, or authorship, what some have called sensegiving (Maitlis and Thomas 2007). Thus nurses were not simply accumulating information and interpreting it; through their sensemaking they were enacting and creating the trajectory narratives that sustained the work.

One of the advantages of storytelling as a mechanism for knowledge-sharing is that stories can be modified for different audiences. Indeed, close examination of nurses' use of trajectory narratives in their everyday interactions with the network actors involved in patient trajectories, reveals that these are not circulated in the same form. Nurses select out and elaborate on those elements relevant to the work purposes of different contributors. So while the work of nurses involves the construction and maintenance of a master trajectory narrative, this provides the resources for the telling of multiple narratives with the particular details adapted according to the needs of the situation. Thus nurses are not simply functioning as a distributed memory system as some have suggested (Bowker *et al.* 2001); in circulating trajectory narratives, they bring about a *translation*. From out of each interaction new translations occur, with questions in one context transformed into answers in another, in an almost continuous flow (Mintzberg 1994). This work is barely perceptible, embedded as it is in the daily interactions with the multitude of actors who move in and out of the care setting.

Knowing what version of a story to tell for different purposes involves the ability to recognise and appreciate others' work purposes and their distinctive ways of understanding the same situation so that the relevant information is prioritised. Boland and Tenkasi (2001) refer to this as perspective-taking. Perspective-taking requires sensitivity to the wider division of labour, the role of others in the activity system and their knowledge requirements. In healthcare, this depends on an understanding of the local role structure, which determines who is responsible for what, rather than interpersonal relationships. This is because when actors are brought together for the purposes of an activity these are often temporary or ephemeral arrangements (Hindmarsh and Pilnick 2002). Although the role formats remain the same, the precise configurations of individuals populating these are variable. Junior doctors, often the first line of contact with nursing staff, are forever changing as they rotate through the services during their training and much specialist input is provided by teams rather than individuals. Moreover, although their use is discouraged in these times of economic austerity, healthcare systems also rely on locum, agency and bank staffs to fill gaps in provision. Nurses invested in these social connections but they could not rely on interpersonal understandings as the basis of organising the work. From a practice perspective, then, knowledge of the role structures relevant to the local ecologies in which nurses worked was an important immaterial artefact through which they accomplished their knowledge mobilisation work.

Taken as a whole, then, nurses fulfilled a central function in creating and circulating the knowledge necessary to support healthcare delivery. Through these largely invisible processes nurses accomplished the momentary 'stabilisations' of trajectory narratives that enabled concerted action. But these were always short-lived agreements; trajectories are constantly on the move and the associated narrative continuously under revision.

Challenges

Creating a working knowledge was not without its challenges. Despite the centrality of handover for the purposes of circulating trajectory narratives, I observed staff complaining about the quality of its content.

> Night Staff Nurse: 'This was not handed over, I read it in the notes, but apparently she's had a five week history of epigastric pain.'

> Staff Nurse: 'They mentioned the cubicle but they failed to tell me that he has shingles!'

Furthermore, nurses could misunderstand the content of handover, or record information incorrectly.

> Coordinator said that one of the staff nurses was having a meeting with a senior nurse and the ward manager this afternoon to discuss an error she has made. This entailed giving medical staff incorrect information about a patient's resuscitation status. The nurse had said that a patient was not for resuscitation when they were. Coordinator said this had happened twice with the same staff nurse. It is possible that she muddled up patients in adjacent beds. Coordinator seems to think that she may have entered the wrong information on her handover sheet. [...] I observed that healthcare professionals appear to be heavily dependent on oral information and make highly consequential decisions on this basis, venturing that in an ideal world nurses would be checking the

record. Coordinator: 'You're too busy. Usually the first time you look at the notes is when you are writing your entries at the end of the day.'

As this last extract indicates, important as this was, consulting the medical notes could be difficult to fit around other demands of the role. Access was a problem because the patient record was often in use by others and locating the relevant information could be time-consuming and entries difficult to decipher.

Deputy Ward Manager: 'We haven't got time to read the notes, so I check on here ((handover sheets)).'

Staff Nurse ((Theatre Recovery)) spends some time leafing through the patient's notes to put together a picture of what has happened to him. Turning the pages, he says that we will probably find that the patient is 'a bit of a one'. Many of the notes are unintelligible and some are contradictory. For example, the Critical Care Unit discharge summary which is a typed document claims he was admitted in April whereas his handwritten medical notes point to a May admission. Together Staff Nurse and I scrutinise some particularly challenging handwriting from an entry made in the Emergency Unit. Only the odd word can be deciphered.

Attending ward rounds was also testing. Multiple teams often arrived at the same time and so nurses had to make choices about where to position themselves. The following extract comes from field notes made on the Surgical Assessment Unit.

08:20 – Suddenly the unit is awash with doctors: some in suits, others in scrubs. There is also a smattering of nurse practitioners. They all arrive at once and it is only the sheer volume of people on the unit which points to this being multiple teams rather than a large single one. Commenting on the challenges of all the doctors arriving simultaneously, Coordinator later informed me that I had witnessed four teams arriving together: medicine, ENT, surgery and urology.

Even though nurses had an important role as a central information source for the purposes of organising healthcare work, they frequently had to adjust their practices and work flexibly around others in order to fulfil this function. How far this reflected the complexity of the field of work or the differential power of ward managers to negotiate satisfactory arrangements with medical colleagues is uncertain, but evidently an issue worthy of further consideration. It was also the case that on units where the coordinator attended the ward rounds, they were frequently required to address other matters. The following field note was made on the Cardiac Surgery Intensive Care Unit.

We move to bed 4. Coordinator is called to the phone and I am faced with the dilemma of whether to stay with the ward round or follow her. I stay with the round. Anaesthetist is talking to a dietician who is seated at the end of the bed completing her notes. Coordinator returns to the round, but is interrupted a few minutes later by a nurse who has concerns about a blood gas result. The ward round discussion continues and includes topics such as whether prescribing Phenytoin and Erythromycin together is contraindicated, whether the patient needs haemofiltration. As this discussion is taking place, the coordinator who has rejoined us, notices a woman with a clipboard standing in the middle of the unit and she 'peels off' once again.

As I have argued, outside of formal coordination events, the principal mechanism through which network actors were enrolled in an individual trajectory was the narrative translations and stabilisations accomplished in the multiple interactions woven through the fabric of healthcare work in which nurses acted as a central information resource. Yet while ensuring communication flows was an important part of the nursing habitus (Bourdieu 2000), others were less diligent. Nurses complained that doctors attending to patients often failed to inform them directly about changes to their management and relied on nurses to consult the medical record.

> Coordinator shows me another set of patient's notes which read 'two more antibiotics, home tomorrow and review by consultant'. Coordinator explained that some of the doctors come to see patients and don't speak to the nurse and so the only way of finding out what is going on is to check the notes. She said the other morning a lady had been written up for a transfusion and the first the nurses knew about it was that there was a slip in the notes. On this occasion someone found it and the lady had the transfusion on time. She said this was a common occurrence and 'then they want to know why someone hasn't had what is required'.

The nurses in the study site adopted different ways of working for the purposes of knowledge mobilisation. One model, which was consistent with the ideals of named nursing,[4] was for the nurse caring for patients clinically to be the repository and primary author of the trajectory narratives. In another model, this function was distributed between the nurses responsible for direct care and the ward coordinator. A third model entailed the whole nursing team operating as a single actor, such that all had an overview of every trajectory on the unit. The nurses I shadowed whose work required them to circulate through a number of ward areas all expressed a preference for the second and third of these models, arguing that while the named nursing model was a good fit with professional ideals, it was impractical for the purposes of the ongoing work, as the responsible nurse might be unavailable and others would be unfamiliar with the trajectory in question.

LIVERPOOL JOHN MOORES UNIVERSITY
LEARNING SERVICES

Back at the other end of the room the Specialist Nurse Practitioners (SNP) are now complaining about the system of patient allocation at night and how, when they arrive on the ward, they are frequently greeted by a nurse who says that 'it is not my patient'. The SNPs are bemoaning the absence of anyone who is in overall charge of the ward. The nurses only have handover on their patients and there is no overall coordinator. I can see why a coordinator would not be necessary at night as there is not a lot to coordinate but I understand the appeal of this role from the SNP's perspective.

Patient Access Nurse said that she preferred working with the wards that have a coordinator and became frustrated when she approached someone with a query only to be told 'Sorry they are not my patient'. She said that when she was working on the wards everyone would have a handover for every patient and that there was a culture of everyone having an overview of activity. In some areas there is a return to this, but in others, named nursing still dominates the organisation of the work.

Discussion

As I described in Chapter 1, in recent history nursing has increasingly come to understand its contribution to society in terms of its care-giving work, and this has been widely understood as underpinned by a distinctive holistic bio-psycho-social approach. Nursing theories and models emphasise the importance of the relationship between nurse and patient such that the clinician might know them as a 'whole person', with some maintaining that it is through the establishment of such healing associations that nursing becomes a therapy in its own right. The more phenomenological aspects of this vision of nursing practice have not been received uncritically (Salvage 1992) and while compassion has been in the forefront of the minds of many people in recent years, it is by no means clear whether patients or nurses want the emotionally intimate relationships so often held up as the ideal. Yet 'knowing the patient' has nevertheless remained an important element of nurses' professional identity and central to practitioners' sense of competence (Allen 1998). My findings indicate that nurses do indeed operate holistically and this appears to be unique to the profession. But this is a rather different holism from that which is commonly assumed; it is a holism founded on the oversight of the whole trajectory of care. In this version, 'knowing the patient' is less about emotionally intimate relationship-building and more about keeping abreast of the diverse constellation of actors, actions and materials that comprise an individual's trajectory of care. Research on collaborative work has identified that different kinds of awareness are necessary to support practice and the generation and circulation of trajectory narratives affords nurses 'activity awareness' for the patients for whom they are responsible. Whereas action awareness relates to information about short-term tasks (Hindmarsh and Pilnick 2002, 2007), activity awareness refers to an awareness of an evolving activity over time (Paul and Reddy 2010). As far as the ongoing management of patient care was concerned, nurses displayed and operated with a unique care trajectory awareness which was unavailable to others. As we have seen, however, nurses come to know the patient through interaction with a complex network of actors – people and artefacts (also, see May 1992). Rendering nurses' knowledge mobilisation work visible brings into view the extent to which these impede or facilitate their work and what might be necessary to better support this aspect of the nursing function. When nurses cannot attend the ward round, or keep being called away, additional effort is needed to establish whether decisions have been taken that are consequential for trajectory management if omissions or discontinuities of care are to be avoided. It is also the case that the home-grown systems that nurses have developed to support their practice are increasingly the target of 'improvement' initiatives, which reveal a profound lack of understanding of the work they claim to support, and carry the risk of unintended negative consequences.

Shift handovers are one of the process modules in the UK National Health Institute for Innovation's Productive Ward Series. Viewed through the prism of Lean management techniques (Womack *et al.* 1990), nursing handover has been criticised for being insufficiently focused and in need of reengineering to streamline the process. Debates about the quality of nursing handover have a long history. Observers from within the profession have underlined its ritualistic quality and the dominance of medical rather than nursing concerns (Ekman and Segesten 1995; Payne *et al.* 2000). Criticism has also been levelled at the time taken in the repetition of information that could be obtained from other sources (McMahon 1990; Sherlock 1995; McKenna 1997). Common to all these views, is an understanding of the purpose of handover as the concise transmission of nursing information (King's Fund 1983; Odell 1996; Miller 1998). Seen from the perspective of nurses' knowledge mobilisation work, however, handovers take on a different hue. Their so-called medical focus makes sense when they are understood as a mechanism for circulating trajectory narratives as part of nurses' organising work rather than as a process for handing over discrete information on clinical nursing care. Furthermore, their worth is not in functioning as a backup to poorly maintained nursing records as some have claimed (Hardey *et al.* 2000), but in transmitting information which is not readily available in formal documentation. There is some evidence that even when the concerns are exclusively biomedical, information on the evolution of an illness trajectory is as relevant to handover as proximal information (Atkinson 1995; Cabitza *et al.* 2005). Thus, to understand handover as a mechanism for transmitting information about nursing care is to miss the point and there are very real dangers in so-called improvement interventions which attempt to strengthen this function and expunge extraneous and supposedly redundant information. Moreover, as we have seen, trajectory narratives are co-created at nursing handover, and thus innovations which aim to achieve efficiencies and reduce staff overlap at shift change through, for example, pre-recorded handover may have unintended consequences.

Munkvold *et al.* (2006) describe an intervention designed to reduce the redundancy thought to characterise nursing handover and offer a salutary lesson. Practice in the study site shifted from a conventional format in which nurses each handed over their own patients to the whole team, to one in which nurses checked the electronic patient record for the patients they had been allocated and then discussed any queries with the person they were taking over from. Rather than the planned change, these authors discovered that: (a) nurses started to arrive early for their shift so that they could renegotiate the patients they had been allocated (previously this was decided after the handover had taken place); (b) the oncoming shift all sitting down after handover on their allocated patients and sharing the information with each other; and (c) the introduction of a whole new system – a weekly written summary of the patient's care as the information gleaned from the electronic record did not include the narrative account of individual progress. What was also lost under the new system was the dialogue between the reporting nurse and those coming on shift, so the interpretative elements necessary to understanding were missing.

In a similar vein, at Parklands, a number of the units had introduced Patient Status at a Glance White Boards (PSAGWB) as part of 'Transforming Care', a regional adaptation of the UK National Health Institute for Innovation's Productive Ward Series. PSAGWBs are an example of visual management and grounded in the belief that making issues more visible provides a shared field of operations (Grief 1991). Communications boards are often used in Lean environments to aid team decision-making by displaying relevant, up-to-date information. In healthcare, at ward and unit level, white boards have been used for many years to indicate bed occupancy. However, PSAGWB are designed to be more than a bed board. They are intended to be a central resource where all vital information is located including: patient vital signs scores, discharge planning progress, patient safety and risk indicators, dietary information and referrals to allied health professionals. The purpose is to make information on a patient's status clear to those who need it and reduce the number of times nursing staff are interrupted by queries from other healthcare providers.

In many ways PSAGWBs are well-aligned with the tools developed by nurses to support their organising work. Thus much of the information replicates that which featured in trajectory narrative plot summaries. The main difference, however, is that PSAGWBs made this publically available. PSAGWBs were normally centrally located at the Nurses' Station and undoubtedly provided a focal point for knowledge-sharing. Personnel attending the ward typically stopped at the PSAGWB as the first port of call and for some the information appeared to be fit for purpose. However, it is also the case, that having studied the PSAGWB, many would also consult nurses about the detail. There were several reasons for this I think. First, one could not be certain of the currency of the information. Healthcare environments are fast-flowing and nurses had to work hard to ensure the information was up-to-date; it often wasn't. Unlike the plot summaries that nurses carried around in their pockets and which could be readily revised, it was necessary to leave the clinical areas in order to update the PSAGWB. So there was inevitably a lag between a change in the patient's status and this being recorded on the white board. Second, it was also the case, that consistent with many quality improvement initiatives, each unit had adapted PSAGWBs for its own purposes. For reasons of patient confidentiality much of the information was conveyed using a singular complex system of symbols in different locales. While localisation is widely believed to encourage ownership of quality improvement interventions and is positively promoted by leaders in the field, for those who circulated multiple wards, it was very difficult to understand anything other than the most obvious information and many needed an interpreter to make sense of the content. Indeed, in some settings, even the local staff did not understand all aspects of PSAGWB content.

Issues of currency and localisation are not insurmountable. But even if these challenges could be overcome, it is also the case that PSAGWBs are based on a script[5] which assumes that the challenge of information-sharing in healthcare is one of access and availability. From an ANT perspective, they are designed to be intermediaries.

> An intermediary [...] transports meaning or force without transformation: defining its inputs is enough to define its outputs.
>
> (Latour 2005: 39)

But as I have argued, when nurses circulated knowledge for the purposes of ongoing patient management, they were not simply accumulating information and transmitting it in an unmodified form; they drew on their clinical and organisational knowledge to interpret, translate and contextualise information for different purposes and for multiple stakeholders. In creating a working knowledge, nurses operated as mediators; they 'transform, translate, distort, and modify the meaning or the elements that are supposed to carry' (Latour 2005: 39).

To assume that PSAGWBs can substitute for nurses is an immense underestimation of the complexity of nurses' knowledge mobilisation function. Indeed they may actually *increase* the work of nurses. PSAGWBs require updating in response to changes in a patient's status arising from decisions taken at the bedside or in interaction with healthcare providers. Much of the information will first be recorded as plot summaries and thereafter transferred to the PSAGWB, creating another step in the process. Furthermore, whereas nurses' plot summaries are private backstage artefacts, PSAGWBs are front-stage technologies. Having a neatly presented PSAGWB was an important signifier of a well-run ward and their ongoing maintenance was an additional demand on nurses' time.

The distinction between intermediaries and mediators is crucial for understanding the limitations of PSAGWBs in supporting knowledge-sharing and calls into question how far they are able to relieve nurses of their knowledge mobilisation work. These observations resonate too with some of the debates in the field of computer supported cooperative work about the types of information system needed in different work contexts. These have centred on the notion of a common information space (CIS) (Schmidt and Bannon 1992), a concept introduced as an alternative approach to workflow models for supporting collaborative activity. Central to this idea is the observation that for information to be shared it has to be extracted from one person's work context and reformulated by means that display its relevance for others. The same information may thus be used by a number of people in different ways. The concept of CIS is supposed to designate both the material carriers of the information, i.e. the representation of the information, and the meaning attributed by actors to these representations (Bossen 2002). The value of the concept is that it relates information use to the activities that are conducted through it. A major preoccupation of work in this field has been with the features of CIS necessary to support knowledge-sharing in diverse work environments (Bossen 2002). Bannon and Bødker (1997) argue that a CIS should be both 'open' and 'closed'; open in the sense of information being interpretatively flexible and closed in the sense of information being portable across practice boundaries. Rolland *et al.* (2006) argue that this characterisation is akin to Latour's (2005) notion of an 'immutable mobile', a term coined to refer to artefacts that are shared across heterogeneous contexts but maintain a relatively stable meaning. This is precisely the intermediary function inscribed in PSAGWBs. Drawing on empirical research in a major international gas and oil company, Rolland *et al.* (2006) suggest that in heterogeneous work contexts, where knowledge-sharing and negotiating common understanding are more fluid, then the key features of CIS are their *malleability* and *momentary* character. They argue for a more dynamic conceptualisation of CIS:

> Rather than focusing on immutable mobiles then, we submit a conceptualization [...] [that] underscores the mutability of objects. Objects are changing – in content, but also in its surrounding network of relationships – constantly.
>
> (Rolland *et al.* 2006: 498)

There are self-evident parallels here with the dynamic status of patient trajectory narratives. In healthcare, where work is widely distributed, understanding of the patient is fragmented and partial and the work is constantly evolving, rather than immutable mobiles such as PSAGWBs, knowledge-sharing requires a 'mutable immobile'; an information source in the sites of care through which knowledge flows around the patient are mediated and stabilised to enable concerted action, and it is nurses who meet this need.

The concept of CIS has been much debated with some increasingly questioning its usefulness (Bannon 2000). Part of the problem I suggest is that thinking in this field has been dominated by the desire to better understand the role of computers in supporting information-sharing in the workplace. While there has been recognition that human actors can facilitate the operation of a CIS by helping both the producers and consumers to package and subsequently interpret information (Bannon and Bødker 1997), none have accorded human actors the central information-sharing function, as in the case of nursing. When we move human agents centre stage, it also becomes necessary to recognise that the work being done is not the maintenance of a space in which information is held in common, but a space in which singular working knowledge(s), that is, stabilised, situated translations, are generated according to the purposes at hand.

Conclusions

There is a prevailing view in organisational studies that knowledge holds organisations together (Brown and Duguid 1998). In this chapter I have examined the work that nurses do in creating a working knowledge to support the practical accomplishment of healthcare. Nurses' knowledge mobilisation work affords them a unique 'activity awareness', which is encapsulated in trajectory narratives which are revised, updated, circulated and translated for different purposes. There is a growing recognition that the notion of narratives is a useful concept in helping us to understand the reasoning processes, interaction and information-sharing in healthcare settings. Narratives are a workable medium for representing knowledge that is time and context dependent and often uncertain and ambiguous as well (Mønsted *et al.* 2011). As I have argued, the medical record is increasingly complex, fragmented and its content oriented to its archival functions rather than supporting everyday work practices. At no place in the formal record is it possible to readily access the current status of an individual's trajectory of care and no other health providers take responsibility for maintaining this overall activity awareness. New mechanisms of visual management attempt to bridge this gap, but these are founded on the assumption that the challenge of knowledge-sharing is one of access and availability, whereas I have argued that successful knowledge mobilisation in healthcare requires translation. It is through the creation and circulation of trajectory narratives that nurses create a mechanism through which the information about an overall trajectory of care is kept in play and then made relevant to individuals' activities in the context of their work. While nurses are the central actors who keep in view the master trajectory narrative, this is always under construction. In their telling, trajectory narratives are always short-lived temporary stabilisations. Somehow healthcare systems function despite this fluidity because the mediating work nurses do keeps multiple shifting visions of the patient and their care in circulation in order for work to proceed. Focusing on nurses' knowledge mobilisation work has also shed light on the profession's claim to practice 'holistically'. Holism, I argue, can best be understood as an organisational rather than an individual phenomenon. While others are increasingly identified with the limited scope of their own specialism, nurses represent not only nursing, but the whole trajectory of care.

Notes

1 These observations have their roots in the notion of 'distributed cognition' (Schutz 1964; Cicourel 1974). As Hutchins (1995) has observed, the social and temporal organisation of cognitive activity outweigh the frequent preoccupation with individual intelligence or cognition in accounting for performance. This underscores the point that organisations can have an important influence on a group's use of cognitive strategies and that to create a satisfactory account of differential human performance, researchers must shift their focus from the cognitive properties of individuals to studies of groups in natural settings (Cicourel 1990).

2 The content of handover varied depending on the features of the trajectory that were relevant to the unit in question. So the trajectories that circulated in acute specialist areas such as intensive care were rich in technical and biomedical details (Carmel 2006) whereas, in the non-acute settings they contained more social and psychological content.

3 Blister packs are a device for dispensing medications when individuals are on complex drug regimes.

4 Named nursing is a derivative of primary nursing, a model of nursing practice in which an individual named nurse is responsible for the management and coordination of a patient's nursing care from the point of admission to discharge.

5 Actor network theorists maintain that formal tools embody assumptions (a script) about the world into which the tool will be inserted. For example, a door presupposes that human actors will open and shut it, if it is to do the job of closing a hole in the wall.

References

Albolino, S., Cook, R. and M. O'Connor (2007). 'Sensemaking, safety, and cooperative work in the intensive care unit.' *Cognition, Technology and Work* 9: 131–137.

Allen, D. (1998). 'Record-keeping and routine nursing practice: the view from the wards.' *Journal of Advanced Nursing* 27: 1223–1230.

—— (2009). 'From boundary concept to boundary object: the politics and practices of care pathway development.' *Social Science & Medicine* 69: 354–361.

—— (2010a). 'Care pathways: an ethnographic description of the field.' *International Journal of Care Pathways* 14: 47–51.

—— (2010b). 'Care pathways: some social scientific observations on the field.' *International Journal of Care Pathways* 14: 4–9.

Armstrong, D. (1983). 'The fabrication of nurse-patient relationships.' *Social Science & Medicine* 17(8): 457–460.

Atkinson, P. (1995). *Medical Talk and Medical Work: The Liturgy of the Clinic.* London, Sage.

Bannon, L. (2000). Understanding common information spaces in CSCW. Workshop on Cooperative Organisation of Common Information Spaces. Technical University of Denmark.

Bannon, L. and S. Bødker (1997). Constructing common information space. Proceedings of the European Conference on Computer Supported Cooperative Work ECSCW'97 Lancaster, UK, Dordrecht: Kluwer.

Barber, N. (2005). 'The pharmaceutical gaze – The defining feature of pharmacy?' *Pharmaceutical Journal* **275**(7358): 78.

Berg, M. and G. Bowker (1997). 'The multiple bodies of the medical record: toward a sociology of artefact.' *The Sociological Quarterly* **38**(3): 513–537.

Boland, R.J. and R.V. Tenkasi (2001). Communication and collaboration in distributed cognition. *Coordination Theory and Collaboration Technology*. G.M. Olson, T.W. Malone and J.B. Smith. New Jersey, Lawrence Erlbaum Associates, Publishers: 51–66.

Bossen, C. (2002). The parameters of common information spaces – the heterogeneity of cooperative work of a hospital ward. Computer Supported Cooperative Work, New Orleans.

Bourdieu, P. (2000). *Pascalian Meditations*. Stanford, CA, Stanford University Press.

Bowker, G.C., Starr, S.L. and M.A. Spasser (2001). 'Classifying nursing work.' *Online Journal of Issues in Nursing* **6**(2). www.nursingworld.org/MainMenu Categories/ANAMarketplace/ANAPeriodicals/OJIN/TableofContents/Volume 62001/No2May01/ArticlePreviousTopic/ClassifyingNursingWork.aspx (accessed 3 May 2013).

Brown, J.S. and P. Duguid (1998). 'Organising knowledge.' *California Management Review* **40**(3): 90–111.

Cabitza, F., Sarini, M., Simone, C. and M. Telaro (2005). When once is not enough: the role of redundancy in a hospital ward setting. GROUP 2005: 158–167.

Carmel, S. (2006). 'Health care practices, profession and perspectives: a case study in intensive care.' *Social Science & Medicine* **62**(8): 2079–2090.

Chen, Y. (2010). Documenting transitional information in EMR. CHI Atlanta, Georgia: 1787–1796.

Cicourel, A.V. (1974). *Cognitive Sociology: Language and Meaning in Social Interaction*. New York, Free Press.

—— (1990). The integration of distributed knowledge in collaborative medical diagnosis. *Intellectual Teamwork: Social and Technical Foundations of Cooperative Work*. J. Galegher, R.E. Kraut and C. Egodo. Hillsdale, New Jersey, Lawrence Erlbaum Associates: 221–242.

Coiera, E. (1997). *Guide to Medical Informatics, the Internet and Telemedicine*. London, Chapman and Hall Medical.

Ekman, I. and K. Segesten (1995). 'Deputed power of medical control: the hidden message in the ritual of oral shift reports.' *Journal of Advanced Nursing* **22**: 1006–1011.

Ellingsen, G. and E. Monteiro (2003). 'Mechanisms for producing a working knowledge: enacting, orchestrating and organizing.' *Information and Organization* **13**: 203–229.

Fitzpatrick, G. (2004). 'Integrated care and the working record.' *Health Informatics Journal* **10**: 291.

Foucault, M. (1973). *The Birth of the Clinic*. London, Tavistock.

Greenhalgh, T., Potts, H.W.W., Wong, G., Bark, P. and D. Swinglehurst (2009). 'Tensions and paradoxes in electronic patient record research: a systematic literature review using the meta-narrative method.' *The Milbank Quarterly* **87**(4): 729–788.

Grief, M. (1991). *The Visual Factory: Building Participation Through Shared Information*. New York, Productivity Press.

Hardey, M., Payne, S. and P. Coleman (2000). '"Scraps": hidden nursing information and its influence on the delivery of care.' *Journal of Advanced Nursing* 32(1): 208–214.

Hindmarsh, J. and A. Pilnick (2002). 'The tacit order of teamwork: collaboration and embodied conduct in anesthesia.' *Sociological Quarterly* 43(2): 139–164.

—— (2007). 'Knowing bodies at work: embodiment and ephemeral teamwork in anaesthesia.' *Organization Studies* 28(09): 1395–1416.

Hutchins, E. (1995). *Cognition in the Wild*. Cambridge, Massachusetts, Bradford Books.

King's Fund (1983). A Handbook for Nurse to Nurse Reporting. Project Paper. London, King's Fund.

Knorr-Cetina, K. (1999). *Epistemic Cultures: How the Sciences Were Made*. Cambridge, Mass, Harvard University Press.

Latimer, J. (2000). *The Conduct of Care: Understanding Nursing Practice*. Oxford, Blackwells.

Latour, B. (2005). *Reassembling the Social: An Introduction to Actor-Network-Theory*. Oxford, Oxford University Press.

Maitlis, S. and T.B. Thomas (2007). 'Triggers and enablers of sensegiving in organizations.' *Academy of Management Journal* 50(1): 57–84.

Manias, E. and A. Street (2001). 'Nurse-doctor interactions during critical care ward rounds.' *Journal of Clinical Nursing* 10(4): 442–450.

May, C. (1992). 'Nursing work, nurses' knowledge and the subjectification of the patient.' *Sociology of Health & Illness* 14(4): 472–487.

McKenna, L.G. (1997). 'Improving the nursing handover report.' *Professional Nurse* 12(9): 637–639.

McMahon, R. (1990). 'What are we saying?' *Nursing Times* 86(30): 38–40.

Miller, C. (1998). 'Ensuring continuing care: styles and efficiency of the handover process.' *Australian Journal of Advanced Nursing* 16(1): 23–27.

Mintzberg, H. (1994). 'Managing as blended care.' *Journal of Nursing Administration* 24(9): 29–36.

Mol, A. (2002). *The Body Multiple: Ontology in Medical Practice*. Durham, NC, Duke University Press.

Mønsted, T., Reddy, M.C. and J.P. Bansler (2011). The use of narratives in medical work: a field study of physician-patient consultations. *12th European Conference on Computer Supported Cooperative Work*, Aarhus, Denmark, Springer.

Munkvold, G., Ellingsen, G. and H. Koksvik (2006). Formalising work – reallocating redundancy. CSCW. Banff, Alberta Canada.

Odell, A. (1996). 'Communication theory and the shift handover report.' *British Journal of Nursing* 5(21): 1323–1326.

Paul, S.A. and M.C. Reddy (2010). 'Understanding together: sensemaking in collaborative information seeking.' *Computer Supported Cooperative Work*: 321–330.

Payne, S., Hardey, M. and P. Coleman (2000). 'Interactions between nurses during handovers in elderly care.' *Journal of Advanced Nursing* 32(2): 277–285.

Power, M. (1997). *The Audit Society: Rituals of Verification*. Oxford, Oxford University Press.

Rolland, K., Hepsø, H.V. and E. Monteiro (2006). Conceptualising common information spaces across heterogeneous contexts: mutable mobiles and side-effects of integration. Proceedings of the 2006 20th Anniversary conference on Computer Supported Collaborative Work, ACM.

Salvage, J. (1992) 'The New Nursing: empowering patients or empowering nurses?' in J. Robinson, A. Gray and R. Elkan (eds) *Policy Issues in Nursing*, Milton Keynes, UK, Open University Press: 9–23.

Schmidt, K. and L. Bannon (1992). 'Taking CSCW seriously: supporting articulation work.' *Computer Supported Cooperative Work (CSCW): An International Journal* 1(1): 7–40.

Schutz, A. (1964). *Collected Papers II: Studies in Social Theory*. The Hague, Martinus Nijhoff.

Seigler, E.L. (2010). 'The evolving medical record.' *Annals Internal Medicine* 153: 671–677.

Sherlock, C. (1995). 'The patient handover: a study of its form, function and efficiency.' *Nursing Standard* 9(52): 33–36.

Strauss, A., Fagerhaugh, S. and B. Suczet (1985). *The Social Organization of Medical Work*. Chicago, University of Chicago Press.

Weick, K.E. (1995). *Sensemaking in Organizations*. Thousand Oaks, London, New Dehli, Sage.

Womack, J.P., Jones, D.T. and D. Roos *et al.* (1990). *The Machine that Changed the World: The Story of Lean Production*. Cambridge, MA, MIT.

3   Articulating trajectories of care

In 2008, Julie Carman was involved in a road traffic accident whilst on a cycling holiday. She suffered injuries to her face, jaw and legs but made a good initial recovery and expected to be back at work within three months.

Three years later she was still undergoing treatment having experienced two further emergency admissions to hospital due to acute cellulitis and sepsis.

A series of 'everyday' communication failures conspired to create delays in her treatment. These led to a slower recovery and in Julie's view were very probably avoidable.

(www.patientstories.org.uk/recent-posts/julies-story-now-available/)

Julie's experience could have been so different if it were not for what she calls, the 'everyday communication failures', which resulted in her not receiving vital antibiotics when needed.

Everyone was very kind to me but no one did anything. A number of medical people said, 'Oh you'll feel better when you get some IV antibiotics', but no one actually gave me any [...] I would say that if they were evaluated individually they would come out fine but I kept falling through the gaps.

From Julie's perspective, it wasn't that individual providers were uncaring; rather, her care fell through the gaps in the system. It is these 'gaps' and the everyday practices through which they are managed that are the focus of this chapter.

Patient care is complex work. Decisions must be made about what should be done, by whom, how, when, where and with what materials, and the more elements involved in the process then the more complicated this becomes. Preventing experiences like Julie's depends on having the right people, with the relevant expertise, equipped with the right knowledge, in the right place, at the right time with the right technologies.

Because patient care is often uncertain, emergent and unpredictable, alignment of all relevant actors in an activity system cannot be taken for granted. Each of the hospital's 'variegated workshops' (Strauss *et al.* 1985) is a distinct constellation of expertise, materials and technologies designed to reflect their particular work purposes and populations served, but in real life people have complex needs which routinely challenge these rational arrangements. Furthermore, while nurses' work is located in the sites of care, others' is more widely distributed. As we saw in the previous chapter, for all their formal structures, large elements of healthcare systems are but loosely coupled and while their contributions may be interdependent at the level of the patient, for much of the time health providers undertake their work in parallel. On the one hand, these arrangements afford actors sufficient flexibility to manage competing demands and respond to the unpredictability of the work. On the other hand, they create very real challenges for service integration. Indeed, despite the complexity of patient care delivery, a curiosity of hospital organisation is that no one is formally charged with responsibility for coordination, although nurses come closest to effecting it, de facto (Glouberman and Mintzberg 2001: 61).

At Parklands, it was largely taken for granted that nurses would organise patient care trajectories. In the daily ebb and flow of personnel through the clinical areas, it was to nurses that junior doctors, allied health professionals and others turned to clarify their contribution and it was nurses who took responsibility for ensuring materials, technologies and tools were available to support activity. Moreover, because healthcare providers came together to align their work infrequently, nurses mediated these relationships. Whether in response to acute, time-critical events, emergent contingencies or simply part and parcel of progressing routine scheduled interventions, nurses made an essential contribution to the alignment and integration of actors necessary for trajectory mobilisation and this largely invisible work was highly consequential for service quality. Following the lead of Strauss *et al.* (1985: 17), I have conceptualised this element of the nursing function as 'articulation work'. Articulation comes from 'articulus', the Latin term for small joint, and refers to the act of connecting things together to allow movement. Articulation is a supra kind of work, requiring skills and resources over and above the immediate task at hand. It is the work that supports the work. As an overall process, articulation takes place everywhere. Everyone has responsibility for fitting together some aspect of their work with somebody else's however minor it may be. Some people are formally assigned to coordinate certain aspects of a course of action, whereas others do a great deal of informal articulation work by virtue of their role (Strauss 1985). This latter kind of work tends to be invisible to rationalised models of organisations (Star and Strauss 1999) and has particular resonance in the case of nursing. In the sections that follow I trace the practices involved in this aspect of the nursing role, the knowledge that underpins it and the barriers to be overcome if nurses are to realise their potential in fulfilling this function.

Bringing the individual into the organisation

Individuals rarely enter healthcare systems with pre-defined needs. A great deal of preliminary work is undertaken to construct a recognisable patient identity around which care can be organised. Nurses make a major contribution to these processes, both at the gateways into the service and through their management of transfers of care (see Chapter 5). From an ANT perspective, this might be understood as a mechanism of 'problematisation', that is the first stage in a process of translation in which a focal actor – in our case the nurse – defines the problem through which others are invited into the network (Callon 1986). The Emergency Unit triage nurse, for example, combined clinical assessment with information from paramedics, patients, family members and documentary sources to establish patients' needs. Several, deemed not to require the expertise of the acute sector, were advised to consult other services; some were referred directly to specialist facilities and others prioritised for medical review as per the departmental protocol. Patients were thereby matched with, and routed towards, distinct activity systems which broadly governed who would contribute to their initial care and the resources required. I observed nurses working at other interfaces undertaking a similar function. A regional centre for certain services, Parklands employed specialist nurses who coordinated access. For example, the cardiac coordinator assessed whether referrals were 'hot or not' and determined the appropriate pathway into the service.

> 'We've got to have a bed and there's the logistics of getting everything lined up'.

Faced with time-critical interventions – such as emergency coronary angiography following a cardiac event or thrombolysis after acute stroke – accelerated translational processes were required in order to have in place the relevant socio-material configurations necessary for action. Individuals must be rapidly enrolled in the organisation on such occasions. Failure to do so costs lives.

Inside the hospital, when an individual is admitted or transferred to an inpatient ward additional effort is required to bring them into the local work organisation. Doctors undertake an initial medical evaluation and set in train a diagnostic and treatment plan, but nurses are instrumental in identifying and initiating requisite actions too. This process is often referred to as a 'nursing assessment', but as I have argued in Chapter 2, this term is somewhat misleading. Nurses typically take a wider view, which extends beyond the requirement for nursing care and is oriented to the potential contribution of others too. The following example relates to an inter-departmental transfer from the Surgical Admissions Unit to the trauma and orthopaedic ward. The coordinator discusses a patient's independence with his wife.

> Coordinator: 'How does he manage with dressing?'
>
> Wife: 'He can only shower and he has a seat; he can manage with my help.'
>
> Coordinator: 'How are you managing?'
>
> Wife: 'It can be a struggle.'
>
> Coordinator: 'We have a social worker on the ward who can advise about sources of support.'
>
> Wife: 'It has been difficult recently as I've pulled this muscle.'
>
> Coordinator: 'Would you like me to make a referral for you?'
>
> Wife: 'Yes please; with my arm as it is it would be very helpful.'
>
> Coordinator: 'We'll start the ball rolling for you.'

It was not unusual for the need for a referral or an intervention to be identified as part of the admissions process and an interesting feature of this extract is that it arises from a routine inquiry designed to ascertain the patient's requirement for nursing support, rather than a formal assessment. As we saw in the previous chapter, nurses accumulate information from a number of different sources and a characteristic of their practice is that knowledge mobilisation and articulation work are interleaved; this is a further feature of the nursing habitus (Bourdieu 2000).

It is well-recognised that normal social interaction is an insufficient basis to support work coordination and the rash of tools to have materialised in healthcare in recent years reflects *inter alia* the desire to better align work activity. At Parklands nurses were largely responsible for assembling the constellation of artefacts intended to support trajectory mobilisation and this was another means through which they brought people into the organisation. In the mountain of standardised forms, charts and checklists available, nurses decided on those indicated in a given case. The stroke coordinator, for example, was at pains to include the stroke pathway in the medical record to ensure patients received the appropriate interventions at the right time. Similarly, when patients were admitted to the Short-Stay Surgical Unit it was nurses who assembled the array of forms and checklists designed to act as prompts for action on the unit, theatre recovery and beyond. How far artefacts succeed in ordering the work in line with their architects' intentions is unclear (Allen 2014). As new institutionalism has shown us, to some extent their organisational value lies as much in their legitimating functions in symbolising the quality of services provided and furnishing a rational account of action (Bittner 1965; DiMaggio and Powell 1983). Moreover, as I argued in Chapter 2, there is a very real tension between the archival and the working patient record and to a considerable extent health providers relied on nurses to generate the narrative knowledge that supported everyday care delivery as formal documentation was inadequate for this purpose. But in so far as the use of such tools was an organisational obligation at Parklands, it was nurses who took responsibility for introducing them into the activity system and this made demands on their time.

Mobilising trajectories

Beyond their role in bringing individuals into the organisation at critical interfaces, nurses worked on an ongoing basis to mobilise evolving trajectories of care. This entailed proactively identifying actions necessary for progress along a planned path and also responsively determining (re)actions indicated by patients' emerging clinical needs and organisational contingencies. While much healthcare can be planned and individual trajectories aligned to formal organisational routines and structures, the distributed nature of healthcare work makes it challenging for contributors to keep track of individual patients. It is also the case that as trajectories evolve, certain actions may be suspended, a given network of actors dissolved and another assembled. All of this must be managed within the temporal constraints of the organisation and actors' competing priorities.

Temporal articulation

Bardram (2000) coined the term 'temporal articulation' to refer to practices which aim to ensure the actions contributing to an activity take place at the appropriate time and in the right sequence. In acute care situations, process-mapping, protocolisation and rehearsal enable participants to be better prepared to ensure that temporal articulation will happen (Draycott *et al.* 2006; Salas *et al.* 2007). Knowing a procedure and one's part in the process makes it possible for healthcare teams to collaborate effectively even if they have not previously worked together. From an ANT perspective, we might think of these as tightly converged actor-networks, where successful translation through formal processes has produced an ordering effect. Networks characterised by a high level of convergence demonstrate agreement as a result of translation and much of the work involved in holding together the relationships between network actors disappears from view; that is, it is black-boxed. But such tightly-coupled assemblages are not available for all eventualities and in such cases it is nurses who have a critical role in mediating the relationships between the constellations of actors required to bring about the alignment necessary for patient care.

Proactive temporal articulation

'Nurses run the place. We are the glue in the system. That requires anticipating people's needs and constantly being two steps ahead.'

Keeping a trajectory on course is skilled and time-consuming work. As we saw in Chapter 2, nurses expend considerable effort in maintaining an overview of patients' ongoing care. But trajectory mobilisation requires more than continuous oversight. It involves predicting how care will unfold so that the necessary arrangements can be made to expedite timely action. This might simply entail prior preparation for planned activity, such as a scheduled operation, requested investigation or forthcoming discharge or ensuring routine interventions are carried out.

She said that in the afternoon she would look at the discharges planned for Thursday and see what needs to be done. 'So I can be proactively phoning the OT ((occupational therapist)) and the physio and getting them to come and do their assessments.'

Night Staff Nurse: '[…] 78 – had laparotomy and abdominoplasty and reversal of Hartmann's ((bowel surgery)). He's eating and drinking. I forgot to look on the computer when his most recent HB ((blood test for haemoglobin levels)) was.'

Staff Nurse: 'Don't worry – I'll look.'

Scheduling activity also required that nurses took into account the temporal constraints of the system. Many services are discontinuous and must be accommodated if delays are not to be incurred. Equipped with a fine-grained understanding of these structures, nurses worked hard to plan ahead (also, see Waterworth 2003). The following field note documents a casual conversation between the coordinator and a staff nurse who were seated together at the Nurses' Station completing paperwork.

Staff Nurse: 'I need to phone the GP ((general practitioner)) about […].'

Coordinator: 'She's going home **Monday** isn't she?'

Staff Nurse: 'Yeah but she's a Warfarin discharge.'

Here, then, the staff nurse vocalises her intention to telephone a GP about a particular patient, and the coordinator registers surprise as the planned discharge date is not for several days. As the staff nurse explains, however, the patient has been prescribed Warfarin, and this requires more advanced notice of the discharge than routine cases. Much of nurses' temporal articulation work involves this kind of anticipatory planning.

'Thinking ahead – that's what it's all about.'

Responsive temporal articulation

Healthcare is dynamic and unpredictable. Because nurses worked at the forefront of evolving patients' needs and the changing shape of the organisation they also performed an important role in responding to these vicissitudes. We might think of this as responsive articulation. To a considerable extent, nurses are the eyes and ears of the organisation and other actors, particularly doctors, depend on their clinical judgement to alert them to the need for an intervention (Allen 1997). The next two extracts are typical examples. The first is taken from observations of a specialist nurse practitioner (SNP) from the Hospital at Night Team who identifies the need for a medical review of a patient whose blood glucose levels are increasing. In the second example, a ward nurse initiates a conversation with the junior doctor about commencing antibiotics on a patient with signs of a urinary tract infection (UTI).

> There is a note in the hospital at night book about a patient's blood sugar levels. The patient has been nil by mouth for 48 hours and is not on insulin but her blood glucose levels are increasing and she has ketones in her urine. The patient tells SNP the doctors have said they will not give her insulin until tomorrow. SNP checks the patient's notes and is not happy. She goes back to the patient and says she will ask the doctors to review her.

> Coordinator: 'Mr X, I think he's got a UTI. He was aggressive in the night. Do you want to start him on anything? [...] His temperature is 38.5, we can do cultures here [...].'
>
> Junior Doctor: 'We could start him on Augmentin ((antibiotic)).'
>
> Doctor writes the prescription.

The need for action might also arise from the ongoing evolution of trajectories. As I have argued, trajectories of care are constantly under revision. Changing understanding of the patient's story can prompt initiation of a new line of work or precipitate the need to locate particular materials. Further to an earlier conversation with a community mental health nurse in which a potential diagnosis of pancreatitis is suggested, in the next extract, the staff nurse initiates blood glucose monitoring on a newly admitted patient.

The HCAs are about to do the BMs. Staff Nurse asks if they can do a 'random BM' on the young man. This relates to the earlier conversation about a possible diagnosis of pancreatitis.

Beyond responding to fluctuating patient needs, nurses also mobilised action in the light of changes in the organisation, such as when a bed unexpectedly became available and a discharge had to be expedited or when a new admission was anticipated. Working flexibly in response to the ebb and flow of organisational life was another facet of the nursing habitus.

Assigning action

Having identified the actions necessary for trajectory progress, it fell to nurses to allocate these to the responsible actor. This could entail a request to undertake a specific task outside nurses' formal scope of practice or a call for specific expertise. It might also involve assigning administrative or housekeeping activities. We might think of this as that part of the translation process known as 'interessement' whereby a focal actor endeavours to convince other actors to accept the definition of their interests. That nurses undertook this work reflects their proximity to patients and their role in maintaining oversight of evolving care trajectories such that they are well-placed to identify necessary actions. As I have argued, many of the actors involved in individual trajectory activity systems worked across a wide area and relied on nurses to notify them if their input was required. Moreover, despite the growing complexity of the healthcare division of labour and the importance of service integration, contributors to a trajectory of care met infrequently and it fell to nurses to make these connections. For example, ward rounds typically were attended by doctors and nurses only and it was taken for granted that nurses would relay decisions that were consequential for the work of others to the appropriate party.

To a considerable extent, the allocation of work was an unremarkable feature of nurses' practice. Indeed, in analysing my data I was drawn to the florid examples of the challenges nurses faced in fulfilling this aspect of their role (see below), but for a long time failed to register the innumerable everyday processes which passed without incident. One reason for this is that for the most part action was assigned through indirect means. As described earlier, when a patient is admitted to a service nurses assemble the relevant coordinating artefacts intended to ensure each contributes their part to an overall process. Moreover, most wards also had some form of doctors' jobs book, a mechanism for referrals to allied health professionals, a social worker's notice board and a messages book for ward receptionists for non-urgent activity, through which nurses assigned tasks. On the admissions units, where rapid patient throughput was a priority, much use was made of central white boards to identify *inter alia* patients required to be seen by which actors, and completed and outstanding actions. In the immediate patient care areas artefacts indicated progress on requested clinical investigations.

> Nurses are writing on the patient notes boxes the observations patients have received or require: ECG, BM, CT. Square boxes are drawn against each and ticked when the task has been carried out.

It was nurses who assumed responsibility for maintaining this information. Artefacts are an important mechanism through which work can be made visible and are useful in a turbulent environment when face-to-face contact cannot be guaranteed and things can be forgotten. They also enabled nurses to keep an oversight of trajectory progress in their areas of responsibility. They are not without their limitations, however, and as we saw in the previous chapter, given a choice, participants preferred to discuss information with nurses.

I have previously interpreted this indirect approach to task allocation as a mechanism for managing the potential for tension when nurses are required to allocate work to those over whom they have no authority (Allen 2001). I suggested that the nursing practice of leaving requests for medical staff rather than soliciting these directly mirrors the intermediary function of the spike in restaurants, which, according to Whyte (1979), acts to mitigate the strains arising from waitresses initiating the work of a higher status colleague, i.e. chefs. On reflection, however, in healthcare these practices appear to arise as much from the practicalities of the work environment as they do sensitivities around negotiating status differentials. First, nurses simply could not guarantee they would be immediately available when relevant actors visited the unit. Second, they juggled several demands and writing a list transfers the task from that of remembering the manifold actions to be undertaken to that of remembering to make an entry. Third, creating a single artefact in which jobs can be accumulated enabled multiple entries by diverse actors which could be checked to avoid repetition. Fourth, a list also conveniently groups all the work for individual actors in one place and obviates the need for them to assess individually each patient under their care.

Having identified the need for an intervention, nurses assessed whether this was urgent or could wait until the responsible actor attended the unit. These were important considerations as many providers worked across a broad terrain and repeated requests to attend the wards disrupted their work organisation. It was important to make such investment in social capital as nurses relied on these relationships in times of difficulty, when trajectories drifted out of control or when they need to work around the system to keep things moving. But such decisions could be finely balanced. The Hospital at Night system at Parklands involved specialist nurse practitioners (SNPs) mediating the relationship between the clinical areas and medical/surgical teams. Wards all used a book to make non-urgent requests, which were screened by SNPs who either addressed the issues themselves or referred them to the medical/surgical teams. Doctors were contacted directly by ward staff for urgent issues. When I shadowed a SNP, we came across an entry relating to a patient with a deteriorating level of consciousness. My respondent observed this to be a serious issue about which the doctor should have been alerted immediately. She reviewed the patient and, having left instructions with the nurses for further observations, requested that the doctors undertake an assessment. Direct patient care was increasingly the responsibility of healthcare assistants and relatively inexperienced nurses and I observed several instances in which senior nurses intervened to escalate action when the need for this had been overlooked by juniors. Indeed, supervisory oversight of junior nurses was becoming an increasingly important and challenging role function across the organisation as the number of senior nurses was reduced to contain costs.[1]

Prioritisation reflected organisational as well as clinical imperatives. A new executive team had recently been appointed at Parklands and a number of my participants pointed to the culture change this had wrought in relation to bed management. As we will see in Chapter 4, pressure on bed utilisation was intense in the hospital and nurses were expected to privilege actions that had implications for expediting patient discharge. Organisational considerations might also require action to be prioritised because that of others depended on it, such as prescription of medication prior to a scheduled specialist investigation, or because of the need to work within wider temporal constraints.

Allocating and prioritising action was integral to the nursing function, but for the reasons outlined, it was relatively invisible. It was in cases of clinical urgency or when professional status boundaries had to be crossed that it was most evident. This is precisely the challenge of studying invisible work; it often remains unquestioned as long as breakdowns do not occur. Yet the case of Julie Carmen illustrates only too clearly what happens when this work is not done, as do the reports of patients reduced to drinking water from flower vases, which emerged in the Mid Staffs Inquiry (House of Commons 2010, 2013). Unremarkable it may be, but allocating action is important work and it was nurses who were the central actors through which the numerous tasks contributing to trajectories of care were mobilised.

Material articulation

Beyond identifying, lining up and assigning tasks, trajectory mobilisation also requires that the necessary materials are available to support the work. I have termed this material articulation. Given that practices are always mediated by artefacts and tools, material articulation is a necessary counterpart to temporal articulation. Research on patient safety in healthcare has repeatedly identified the unavailability of equipment and/or medications as factors that have contributed to catastrophic outcomes in critical incidents (National Patient Safety Agency 2007; BBC 2012; Telegraph Reporters 2012). With their work located in the sites of care, it was nurses who took responsibility for ensuring the accessibility of resources and materials.

One aspect of this work related to the maintenance of the clinical environment. Both through their routine safety checks and their everyday practice, nurses took responsibility for ensuring materials were available when needed. They inspected resuscitation trolleys to make certain equipment functioned and drugs were available and had not expired, assessed the integrity of mattresses for infection control purposes (any punctures representing a risk), and undertook ongoing surveillance of ward equipment and stock levels. They also monitored the availability of materials in relation to anticipated demand. This entailed forecasting the evolution of trajectories of care in the population of patients currently on the unit and planning ahead, taking into account the temporal constraints of the organisation.

> Coordinator: 'Fentanyl – there are only five in the cupboard and I have ordered more. You'll be OK for today.'

> She then lists the patients on the unit with Patient Controlled Analgesia, the main demand for Fentanyl.

> Emergency Unit Coordinator and I spend time checking the mattresses on the trolleys in the corridor. Some of the mattresses are very thin and patients should not be on them for more than 2 hours for tissue viability reasons. She knows she is going to have trolleys in the corridor today and that people may be waiting a long time. We scour the department looking for trolleys with deep mattresses. We bring these into the corridor and take trolleys with thin mattresses into the assessment areas.

> Coordinator bumps into the ward pharmacist on her way to coffee break.

> Coordinator: 'Oh, I decided not to bleep you but we've run out of IV GNT (Glyceryl Trinitrate).'

> Pharmacist: 'I put enough up for 24 hours; have they increased the dose?'

> Coordinator: 'No. My concern is that it's a bank holiday weekend and I don't want to run out.'

In this last example, the nurse draws on her knowledge of the hospital's temporal order and marries this with an understanding of projected patient trajectories in order to ensure the IV GNT will be available. It was not always possible to plan in advance, however, and in such circumstances resources had to be located from other departments. The site coordinators had an important trouble-shooting role locating materials when unexpected contingencies arose.

Site Coordinator said she was often called when someone had a broken bed and had to find a replacement. Whenever she is passing through the tunnels under the hospital she makes a point of looking to see whether beds and mattresses are available.

It was also the case that while most units routinely had in place the appropriate configuration of materials and technologies to support the population of patients they were designed to care for, the imperative to meet singular patient requirements and to use beds flexibly made it necessary to make arrangements for equipment to be sourced elsewhere. Equipment sharing in such circumstances could also entail exchanging the associated technical and organisational knowledge.

> Coordinator: 'There's an ongoing issue with Snowdrop Ward and tracheostomy inner tubes. We sent them over 10 boxes and there's been a bit of miscommunication and some think they are reusable despite us going down and explaining. The other thing they want is to order some and don't know how to go about it.'

Sharing resources was part of the organisational culture and such pragmatic actions were vital for trajectory progression.

Beyond their work in maintaining a functioning clinical environment, nurses often assembled materials to support specific actions. This was necessary in circumstances in which providers were operating under pressures of work, when action was time-critical and, where actors were unfamiliar with the location of resources and equipment. For example, in the acute admissions areas nurses reviewed test results and informed doctors when these became available in order to expedite decision-making. Nurses across the organisation also routinely assembled the materials required to expedite particular work processes, such as medication charts to be updated by doctors or pharmacists, forms to be completed or the equipment required to undertake a procedure. Often this was simply a mechanism for expediting action to ensure temporal articulation of a routine intervention, but in certain circumstances it could be essential for supporting care coordination in acute scenarios. For example, the stroke coordinator was responsible for preparing the field to support thrombolysis, an intervention to be administered within three hours of the onset of a stroke. When a patient was expected, the on-call medical team would be called to the Emergency Unit and the stroke coordinator oversaw the process. This included ensuring certain tasks were undertaken and assembling the requisite materials to support the procedure.

> 'I go to see everything is ready and I draw up the medicines loads and stay with the patient until they are transferred to the Stroke Unit'. [...] This includes ensuring a whole range of things have taken place before

hand because of the risks of bleeding after the procedure: swallow screen, NG tubes, catheterisation etc.

Nurses also had a role in supporting the material articulation of others' practice because of their greater familiarity with the clinical care settings. Considerable work was underway at Parklands to rationalise and systematise individual units and a number of locales had deployed Lean principles to reorganise ward storage areas. It was intended that this would reduce the time spent by nurses searching for supplies and equipment in order that they might spend more time at the bedside. However, given that units were organised along very different lines, these changes did nothing to reduce the dependency of visitors on nursing staff for locating materials.

> The Trauma and Orthopaedics team are hanging around the desk area. One of them is speaking into a Dictaphone and pausing occasionally to verify information from the patient's notes [...]. The doctors are evidently unfamiliar with the ward, in fact at one point one asks 'Where are we?' One is trying to locate a blood request form and wanders up and down the corridor for a bit before asking: 'Are there any nurses on this ward?' His colleague directs him to the desk at the central reception area where all the medical forms are kept.

It might be argued that the work nurses do to assemble the materials necessary to support action is continuing evidence of the so-called handmaiden role, or the 'adjunct work' Celia Davies (1995) has written about, but in pressured environments where many actors operate across diverse settings and lack familiarity with ward practices and layout, it is essential to guarantee activity is undertaken smoothly.

Integrative articulation

In addition to the work that is done to facilitate action, trajectory mobilisation also requires effort to ensure all the different elements cohere. Beyond formal coordinating mechanisms, 'mutual adjustment' (March and Simon 1958) or 'relational coordination' (Gittel *et al.* 2000) is often presented as the process through which workers align their respective contributions in the workplace. But as I have argued, in healthcare, providers directly interact infrequently and nurses have an important role in mediating these relationships. I have called this aspect of their work 'integrative articulation'.

Promoting holistic decision-making

Because nurses operated with an overview of patient trajectories, they had an understanding of the inter-relationships between constituent elements. Cabitza *et al.* (2007) term this 'coordinative awareness', that is, an awareness of the interdependencies in an activity system. Actions that seem entirely reasonable in their own terms might be called into question from a trajectory perspective. In multidisciplinary team meetings, such issues could be discussed explicitly, yet these were intervallic events and outside of these occasions nurses interceded between actors to ensure decisions were undertaken in the context of patients' overall needs. We might think of this element of the nursing function as promoting holistic decision-making.

The need for holistic decision-making was most evident on the ward round, a key coordination event that, in most settings, was attended by doctors and nurses only. Ward rounds were front-stage performances conducted at the bedside and nurses' work in promoting holistic decision-making in this context was extraordinarily subtle. I saw no examples in which nurses openly disagreed with a medical decision; but I observed numerous occasions in which they acted to influence the outcome of deliberations, typically through the provision of additional information. In the following example, the coordinator introduces supplementary information when the doctor is about to make a decision to remove a catheter. The doctor's question – Do you need that catheter? – is addressed to the patient and might reasonably be understood to relate to the narrow subject of urinary functioning, whereas the nurse's intervention points to the relevance of mobility too, a factor the patient is unlikely to take into account in response to the question as expressed by the doctor:

Registrar: 'You're on antibiotics for your chest. Do the nebulisers help?'

Patient: 'Yes they help.'

Junior doctor listens to the patient's chest and says it sounds better. 'We did a chest X-ray recently.'

Patient: 'Sunday.'

Registrar: 'We should check on that; it's been a couple of days. I'll have a chat with Mr [...] about eating and drinking. Do you need that catheter?'

Coordinator: 'He's not very mobile.'

We see similar subtle influencing processes in this second extract. Here the doctor informs the patient he can be discharged home. From the perspective of overall trajectory management, however, medical fitness is only one factor in reaching a discharge decision. The nurse is oriented to this and asks the patient whether he has had a mobility assessment: 'Have you done the stairs?' Although not directly questioning the doctor, her inquiry creates the potential for new information to be brought into play which might have implications for decision-making. Her intervention in this case appears to be prompted by the doctor's last minute reference about the need to check the wound indicating that he has not taken into account all relevant elements of the patient's condition in reaching his initial decision.

Junior doctor: 'We need to check the potassium I think and check the stool and then we can think about getting home. If I can sort out the paperwork you can go today if all's OK. ((The doctor makes as to leave the room and says almost as an afterthought)): How's the wound? I suppose I'd better check' ((Returns and examines the patient's abdomen)).

Coordinator asks the patient: 'Have you done the stairs?'

Patient says he has.

As these extracts illustrate, the means through which nurses achieve holistic decision-making are understated. In neither example does the nurse overtly question the doctors' decision; their contribution is carefully crafted to widen the range of factors to be taken into account in reaching a final judgement. These delicate influencing skills perhaps help to explain the observations made by others about nurses' limited input into decision-making during ward rounds (Latimer 2000; Manias and Street 2001) and it also resonates with a growing body of sociological research which has highlighted the distributed nature of decision-making in healthcare (Bloor 1976; Berg 1992; Rapley 2008; Goodwin 2013). That nurses adopted indirect influencing strategies points to the uncertain authority with which they carry out articulation work. In their front-stage behaviours such as on the ward round they were clearly oriented to the higher status of medicine and acted to reinforce this in front of patients. Whereas in the backstage regions away from the bedside, their interactions with medical staff were more direct.

Resolving anomalies and contradictions

Beyond their work in fostering holistic decision-making, nurses played an important role in resolving anomalies or contradictory elements in trajectories of care. That these disconnections can arise is one of the challenges of the loose coupling that characterises much healthcare work in a context of growing specialisation. Because nurses have oversight of overall trajectory progress and a wider understanding too of the systems and processes through which care is organised, they are well-placed to identify these issues and indeed anticipate potential problems before they arise. In the following example, the nurse contacts a doctor to clarify an earlier instruction to administer a dextrose infusion to a patient with diabetes. The nurse knows that the dextrose infusion was prescribed by the first doctor as a source of energy when it was assumed that the patient would be 'nil by mouth'. Now she is eating it is no longer required, but the nurse has no authorisation to cancel the doctor's request and the doctor has no way of knowing about the subsequent decision by the second medical team.

Staff Nurse makes another call to another doctor to clarify earlier advice about a dextrose infusion and 2 hourly BMs in the light of a decision taken by another team that the patient can eat and drink for now but will be nil by mouth from midnight.

Trajectory integration extended beyond actions to the socio-material configurations necessary to support patient needs. In the next example, the nurse negotiates with the doctor over a drug dosage. She is concerned because the medications do not come in tablet form in the dosage prescribed and the patient, who is about to be discharged home, is unable to break them in half in order to administer the correct dose.

> Staff Nurse: '[…] has gone down to 90 is there any chance you could go to 100 as they don't have 90 tablets and he's got to give them himself.'
>
> Junior Doctor: 'When I increase it, it increases his epistaxis so it's likely to have to come down further.'
>
> Staff Nurse: '80 – they do 80 tabs: OK so I can have a word with the registrar.'

This is a finely wrought judgement in which the nurse draws on her knowledge of the patient and the dose formats of this medication to identify the potential risks involved in discharging the patient home on his current prescription. Such interventions can be highly consequential for medication adherence and yet go largely unnoticed in the cacophony of decisions that shape trajectory management. As we saw in Chapter 2, much of the work that nurses do in making sense of trajectories is triggered by anomalies or discrepancies of some kind. Being alert to these and acting to resolve them was an important mechanism through which trajectories were mobilised.

Facilitating planning

The nursing contribution to ensuring trajectory coherence is threaded through their everyday work and interleaved with their knowledge mobilisation practices. Nevertheless, there is a growing realisation in healthcare of the need for better care integration and that a multidisciplinary approach is an important mechanism through which this can be achieved. Thus in many units, particularly where patients characteristically had complex continuing care needs, ward rounds were supplemented with weekly multidisciplinary meetings which were key fora in which trajectories could be stabilised and all actors brought together to negotiate their respective contributions. Amidst the highly distributed and fragmented arcs of work through which trajectories of care were routinely mobilised, these represented key crystallisation points[2] in which, for a short period, trajectory narratives could be held in common for planning purposes. At Parklands, nurses in specialist roles were emerging as an important force behind these events and in several locales had been instrumental in improving their effectiveness.

LIVERPOOL JOHN MOORES UNIVERSITY
LEARNING SERVICES

Stroke Coordinator said that she felt that the Multidisciplinary Team Meeting had improved in recent years. 'I am happier that we have a good overview and that we have something written down in relation to goals and plans.' She said that she felt that the consultant still talked too much about the medical issues and he needs to say less – not least because he has already discussed these issues on the ward round – and listen to what the therapists have got to say. But 'it's early days and we're getting there'.

Nurses played a key part in initiating and orchestrating multidisciplinary meetings and were forthright in pushing for goal-setting, decision-making and clarification of roles and responsibilities. The following extract is taken from the neuro-rehabilitation team meeting, in which the nurse coordinator pushes for a formal plan.

Neuro-Rehabilitation Coordinator: 'Good morning Mr [...] ((The meeting has already started and the Consultant has arrived late)). Should we plan for discharge if he doesn't need to be here? Does he need a [...] bed?'

Physiotherapist: ((I missed the response))

Neuro-Rehabilitation Coordinator: 'Does he need a Zimmer?'

Physiotherapist: 'No, he's not up on a Zimmer.'

Neuro-Rehabilitation Coordinator: 'If he was at home what would the timescales be for training? Would we bring him back in?'

Physiotherapist: 'We wouldn't need to bring him back in. We could do it as an outpatient.'

[...]

Neuro-Rehabilitation Coordinator: 'Could we have a meeting next Friday to explore where we are and move forward?'

[...]

Consultant: 'He lives on his own?'

Physiotherapist: 'He has a family, but lives on his own.'

Clinical Nurse Specialist: 'He has an ex partner who is still very much involved.'

Neuro-Rehabilitation Coordinator: 'I think he could go. He doesn't need to be here; it's just because of his housing. Does he know what's happening with it?'

Physiotherapist: 'He knows it needs to be done but he doesn't know any more than us.'

Neuro-Rehabilitation Coordinator: 'OK that's it then: fact finding. Who's going to let the social worker know? ((to SN)): Could you contact them and let them know because discharge is imminent. If you let them know then it might galvanise them into action.'

Here, then, the neuro-rehabilitation coordinator takes the lead in establishing relevant information about the status of a patient's trajectory of care. The extract opens with an agreement that the patient no longer needs to remain in hospital and the conversation moves onto discharge planning. The coordinator asks pertinent questions of the physiotherapist about the patient's requirement for a specialist bed and whether he needs a Zimmer frame to mobilise. These are important considerations; if needed these will have to be ordered before discharge. A decision is then taken to set plans in motion and the coordinator charges the staff nurse with responsibility for contacting the social worker to address the housing issues. In this example, the doctor is uncharacteristically passive. Approaching retirement, he was widely perceived to be disaffected and this created specific difficulties in this service. Notwithstanding the singular qualities of this particular case, elsewhere in my notes I made summative observations of the team meetings on the stroke unit and noted how 'both Stroke Coordinator and Discharge Liaison Nurses drive the organisational elements of the meeting and channel and prompt people's thinking'.

Thus, as well as having a leading role in initiating, allocating and aligning action, in progressing patient care, nurses also had an important function in ensuring trajectory integration. The need for this arises because much of healthcare work is loosely coupled. Actions taken by one party for one purpose can be consequential for other elements of care, the responsibility for which lies elsewhere. It is also the case that providers operate with a partial picture of patient needs, determined by their own work purposes. Nurses retain oversight of the evolution of trajectories and mediate these relationships in order to prevent trajectory fragmentation. This entails an understanding of how decisions interact at the level of an individual's clinical care. They were also taking a leading role in multidisciplinary planning processes.

Maintaining progress

Maintaining trajectory momentum involved continuous effort. Medical teams had to be tracked down to establish patient treatment plans, the outcome of investigations followed up and progress on discharge planning arrangements ascertained. Work-a-rounds might also be necessary to circumvent obstacles to progress. When the emergency unit sought to discharge a patient back to his warden controlled accommodation when he did not have his keys, it was the coordinator who 'was phoning the world and his wife' to sort out the problem. When it transpires that the doctors have omitted to prescribe laxatives for a patient to be discharged home, the staff nurse negotiates with the pharmacist for these to be dispensed so as not to delay progress. And when Mrs Green's discharge threatens to be delayed because she requires blister packs, the nurses negotiate with the local Pastor who agrees to give her medicines until these are available. There is a sense in which hospitals need such flexible arrangements in order to cope with the unpredictability and complexity of the work. But centrifugal forces are inherent in this kind of organisational form and trajectories can easily go off course. The mobilisation of trajectories of care required continuous effort to ensure their various elements did not pull apart and it was nurses who performed this function. Their articulation work arose from and was a necessary counterpart to the distributed nature of healthcare work.

Activity system knowledge

The work that nurses do to articulate trajectories of care is closely intertwined with their knowledge creation function and the activity awareness afforded by trajectory narratives (Chapter 2). However, the mobilisation of patient care required other kinds of intelligence too, namely, understanding of the associated activity *system*. This included cognisance of the local role structure and coordinative awareness of interdependencies (Cabitza *et al.* 2007) but also sophisticated clinical, contextual and organisational knowledge. A common but, as yet, unremarked upon feature of trajectory articulation was its reliance on nurses' ability to identify relevant organisational and clinical patterns and match these with the appropriate routines. It has long been acknowledged that routines are an aid to cognitive efficiency and useful for managing complexity. My data indicates that amidst the turbulence of nurses' everyday work, pattern recognition and organisational routines were the principal resources through which trajectories were mobilised. Thus specific *categories* of patient acted as triggers for particular courses of action. One of the coordinators described how it was possible to anticipate patients who would be eligible for continuing care funding ('CHC patients') which allowed the process of referral for beds to be initiated to expedite the discharge process.

> Coordinator said that it was possible to recognise CHC patients early on and they could start to informally make arrangements for their care before a decision was taken that they were medically fit to leave.

Certain *decisions* were also associated with routine lines of work. For example, in the following extract, note how the night staff nurse's observations that 'she's query home today' stimulates the coordinator to list the actions (TTHs, OPA and GP letter) required to expedite the discharge.

Night Staff Nurse: 'She's query home today if her pain is controlled and she has her bowels open.'

Coordinator writes: 'Home, TTHs ((tablets to take home)), OPA ((outpatient appointment)) and GP letter' each with its own red tick box down the left hand side of her handover sheet.

Routines apply to material configurations as well as activity (Bardram and Bossen 2005). So, for example, the announcement of an expected admission to the Intensive Care Unit galvanises action to prepare the field for the patient's arrival.

Clinical Director: 'There's a man on ((surgical ward)) with hospital acquired pneumonia who we're going to have to connect. [...] Which bed space do you want me to admit him to?'

Coordinator: 'He can go into ((bed)) 5. What drugs do you want?'

I missed the Clinical Director's response. Coordinator informed the nurse in the area and began checking the equipment, drawing up drugs and labelling them. [...] Other nurses move into action, one covers the bed with paper sheets and a 'pac slide' ((a device for moving patients)), another is running through IV bags and connecting these to equipment. At one point five people are contributing to the preparations; each seems to know what they're doing and the division of labour occurs without any explicit discussion. [...] Coordinator then checks the drugs she has drawn up with the nurse caring for the patient. Another nurse says: 'I have checked the trolley and its all fine'. ((She was referring to the trolley with all the ventilator equipment on it)).

Different *clinical presentations* were also associated with discrete interventions. This next field note is from handover on the Cardiac Surgical Intensive Care Unit. The nurse is accounting for the care of a female patient who has been slow to recover from an anaesthetic. Having outlined the actions taken to establish there are no other underlying reasons for the patient's sluggish progress, the nurse notes that her clinical presentation suggests that Lasix might be indicated ('She has a colloid balance of 1.8 and I think a crystalloid balance of [...]'). She is, however, at pains to stress that she raised this with the anaesthetist who instructed her to review the position in the morning. Here, then, the nurse demonstrates that she has noted and responded to the clinical presentation of the patient, identified the appropriate intervention, contacted the responsible actor, but was advised to wait before acting.

She has a colloid balance of 1.8 and I think a crystalloid balance of [...] and I did ask the anaesthetist about Lasix but he said leave it until the morning. But I did ask.

The nurse clearly is oriented to background assumptions about her responsibility to intervene in such circumstances and the departure of this patient's trajectory from the normal course of action is accountable. Indeed when decisions or lines of action did not follow recognised paths, nurses were observed to seek clarification. In the next extract the nurse knows that Frusemide is often administered when a patient is in receipt of a blood transfusion and in this case it has not been prescribed.

> Staff Nurse: 'Do you want him to have Frusemide between bloods?'
>
> Doctor: 'I won't bother with him. He's in a negative balance anyway.'
>
> Staff Nurse: 'OK just checking.'

Although there are immeasurable incidents in which the relationship between pattern recognition, the application of a routine and subsequent action appear to proceed in a linear fashion, as these last two examples reveal, patterns and routines do not determine patient care in a straightforward way. One way of thinking about this relationship is in terms of the distinction between the 'ostensive' and the 'performative' aspects of routines (Feldman and Pentland 2003). The ostensive element of a routine is the abstract pattern that participants use to guide, account for and refer to specific performances. The performative aspect refers to the actual instantiation of the routine enacted by specific people, at specific times in specific places. Having identified the relevant pattern as a trigger for action, nurses use the ostensive aspect of routines to make sense of and identify the network of actors necessary for the mobilisation of trajectories but the enactment of routines is left to the responsible provider. While nurses have trajectory awareness they do not share the specialist knowledge of activity system members, but by deploying the ostensive routines of the activity systems with which they are familiar they bring this expertise to patients. In this way then, lines of action are mobilised without these needing to be specified on each occasion, timely interventions can be made and errors and omissions avoided. Through their practice of matching patterns with organisational routines nurses were an important engine of trajectory mobilisation.

With the extension of management logic and clinical governance across developed healthcare systems, there has been considerable debate about the role of standardisation in healthcare. Yet discussion of the pluses and perils of these trends largely overlooks the central role of routines as mechanisms that support work organisation. Indeed as Glouberman and Mintzberg (2001: 71) argue, 'professional work in the healthcare system is not about open-ended problem solving so much as about closed-ended pigeonholing – slotting the condition of the client into one or more of the available procedures of the provider'. This, they argue, is one of the great strengths of healthcare systems but also one of its weaknesses. Glouberman and Mintzberg argue that while such mechanisms of coordination work more or less successfully for closely-bounded clinical procedures such as surgery, they are less well-suited to wider elements of healthcare provision. Thus, they argue, that: 'activities are pigeon holed into pat categories and then assumed to be coordinated by virtue of what everyone is supposed to know about the work of everyone else [...]. Even to the extent that these pigeon holes work in medicine – which is becoming less true – it works less well beyond medicine, and so this assumption leads to all kinds of duplications, misunderstandings, and mistakes' (ibid.: 72). While these observations are prescient, my data suggest that trajectory coordination does not depend on everyone knowing about the work of everyone else, it depends on nurses mediating these relationships. That this is absent from Glouberman and Mintzberg's characterisation of healthcare is unsurprising given what we know of the invisibility of the nursing contribution and insights from new institutionalism of the loose coupling between formal organisational structures and everyday work processes.

There is an apparent contradiction between the observation here that nurses combined pattern-recognition and organisational routines to mobilise trajectories and my assertion in Chapter 2 that formal tools, such as care pathways, did not feature prominently in their everyday practice. This is because the routines nurses deployed were largely taken-for-granted knowledge. Routines can be held in 'procedural memory' and become part of organisational members' tacit understandings (Cohen and Bacdayan 1994). Moreover, as Feldman and Pentland (2003) argue, the artefactual element of a routine (such as pathways) should be considered separately from the ostensive and performative elements. Indeed we might go further, and conceptualise the ostensive element of routines as comprising of material and immaterial or psychological (Vygotsky 1978) elements. Material artefacts such as integrated care pathways are important in specifying the routines involved in idealised pathways of care, and important signifiers of quality within the organisation. But in their everyday practice, the routines nurses deployed were largely immaterial. Thus, routines comprise abstract understandings, specific performances and a whole host of associated artefacts that are not always in alignment and we should be cautious about using one element to characterise any of the others (Pentland and Feldman 2005, 2008).

Challenges

Despite the importance of trajectory articulation for the quality of patient care and the efficiency of the organisation, nurses faced many challenges in fulfilling this function. As I have argued, nurses' practice was underpinned by activity system knowledge and this was highly effective for coordinating activities in the clinical micro-systems (Mohr and Batalden 2002) with which they were familiar. But the growing number of outliers in the ward areas, that is, patients placed in beds outside of the service responsible for their care, made this work more difficult.

> The problem with outliers is that the staff don't know what's going on with them until they are seen. (Patient Access Nurse)

Anticipatory planning was challenging as nurses did not have access to relevant patterns and routines and it was difficult to allocate action without familiarity with the working practices of the different specialists involved. In caring for patients who had conditions with which they were not conversant, one might also aver that nurses were less well positioned to detect clinical signs that signalled the need for an intervention, although this is a logical rather than an empirical inference.

Nurses relied heavily on their procedural memory to articulate action and did not appear to deploy formal pathways in their everyday practice. Yet while this undoubtedly reduced transaction costs which benefited the organisation, it also created difficulties when these were superseded by new guidance. On the colorectal ward, a new 'Enhanced Recovery after Surgery' pathway was being implemented and the consultant complained that junior doctors were not prescribing the intravenous infusion as per the agreed regime. It emerged that doctors were being guided by nurses who, rather than directing them to the pathway, were drawing on old routines.

> Staff Nurse: 'Mr [...] has brought up the issue of IVs again. They're writing these up 8 hourly when it should be 62.5ml per hour if they are on enhanced recovery.'
>
> Coordinator: 'Is this a nursing issue?'
>
> Staff Nurse: 'Well the girls are getting them to write them up on nights.'

This extract makes explicit the blurred lines of responsibility here. The coordinator questions whether this is a nursing issue; strictly speaking, it is not. However, the staff nurse orients to the real world of practice where articulation depends on the direction of nurses and on this occasion they were at fault.

Specialisation in healthcare is growing and, for a whole range of reasons, providers increasingly work with a tightly circumscribed view of the categories of patient on which their skills might be brought to bear. Medical teams often were unable to agree who was responsible for a given patient and when such deliberations were protracted, trajectory progression could be delayed.

> Coordinator: 'She came in under us but was referred to Neuro and referred back again and no one has seen her. She's been in 8 days.'

While they were not responsible for resolving these disputes, nurses were often observed to exert pressure on medical teams to make a decision, but their power to influence was limited.

Although nurses played an important role in allocating work in response to the evolving status of trajectories, their formal jurisdiction imposed certain constraints on their practice. For example, the anaesthetic pre-assessment nurses, while recognised to possess advanced clinical skills that permitted them to assess patients' suitability for anaesthesia, were not formally mandated to request additional investigations. This was the responsibility of anaesthetists. With no resident clinician in the department, however, it was difficult to make contact with the responsible actor and the nurses worked around the system by making the request and signing on behalf of the anaesthetist. That nurses informally blur the boundaries of their practice in order to ensure the smooth running of the service is well-recognised (Allen 2001) and there were numerous other such examples in this particular study, driven by an underlying desire to mobilise action in the interests of patients.

Although nurses were taking a leading role in orchestrating multidisciplinary events, ultimate responsibility for deciding on a patient's suitability for discharge resided with the consultant. I attended a number of multidisciplinary meetings where senior doctors failed to attend which severely constrained the team's ability to reach a decision and plan ahead. It was also the case, that several team meetings on the medical wards were cancelled as the consultant could not be there. This was a clear source of delay in the decision-making required to support discharge planning.

As we have seen, trajectory mobilisation requires actions to be prioritised and this could be for both clinical and organisational reasons. There is a research literature which highlights the difficulties nurses sometimes encounter in persuading those in more senior positions to take action and this can result in a failure to rescue deteriorating patients (Silbey 2009). In this study I did not encounter or hear reports of serious clinical incidents of this kind but it was evident that junior doctors did not always recognise the urgency of organisational imperatives. What looks like a non-urgent task from a clinical perspective, could be hugely consequential for the organisation. Nurses often found it necessary to expend considerable time and energy locating junior doctors to complete their work in order that trajectories of care could be progressed.

> The receptionist and coordinator are getting frustrated as they cannot get one of the junior doctors to answer the bleep. Between them they have bleeped her five times. Coordinator ((to me)): 'We can't get hold of the doctors to come and do the jobs.'

> Bank nurse said that she spent all her time on the phone trying to get hold of the doctors.

At the time of the study an internal survey was underway which required nurses to systematically record when doctors were requested to undertake an activity and for doctors to indicate when this had been accomplished. This, I understand, was an attempt to establish the veracity of nurses' claims that delays to trajectory progress arose from the failure of junior doctors to fulfil their responsibilities. While at one level this was an important achievement on the part of nurses in garnering formal recognition of their organising work, at another, despite deliberate effort, I did not locate one example in which the form had been completed as required!

Implications

In this chapter I have argued that nurses have a leading role in articulating the socio-material configurations necessary for the progression of trajectories of care and have shown the importance of their work for service quality. In some areas, nurses in specialist roles were emerging as a significant force in orchestrating multidisciplinary decision-making, but on the wards nurses' organisational status as care coordinators was ambiguous and they were required to influence the work of a range of healthcare providers over whom they had little formal authority. Previous research has identified the challenges of coordination across functional boundaries in the absence of supervisory responsibility (Clarke and Wheelwright 1992). I have described how, on the ward round, nurses adopted subtle tactics to influence decision-making, rather than tackling these issues directly which potentially limited their influence. Jurisdictional boundaries that got in the way of progress were overcome as far as possible by informal working practices, but the fact that the system continued to function depended on the goodwill of nurses and their preparedness to bend the rules in the interests of patient care. There were also aspects of the system that were more taxing for nurses to circumvent, such as disputes between doctors about responsibility for the care of patients. Finally, at Parklands nurses' role as the eyes and ears of the organisation was becoming increasingly challenging in a context in which senior posts had been reduced which made it more difficult to supervise healthcare support workers and junior nurses who were primarily responsible for direct clinical care.

Trajectory articulation is essential for the quality and safety of patient care and the efficiency of organisations and my findings underline the need for formal recognition of nurses' care coordination role. Not only do nurses need the authority to negotiate with the full range of stakeholders directly to orchestrate care, organisations should also put in place local arrangements to enable nurses to overcome the obstacles and jurisdictional restrictions that prevent them from fully realising their potential in fulfilling this role function. At Parklands, in a number of locales certain nurses were emerging as the lead professional in coordinating complex discharge arrangements and appeared to be accorded the authority to successfully fulfil this function. But these arrangements were aligned with organisational priorities around discharge planning rather than trajectory management more widely.

Conclusions

In conventional understandings of healthcare work, it is medicine that is viewed as the principal actor and the decisions made by doctors are unquestionably consequential for trajectory progress. Yet when we scrutinise the invisible work of nurses, it becomes clear that every day through a multitude of seemingly unremarkable activities, it is nurses who shape and reshape patient care and who provide the energy that sustains trajectory momentum. Their work is essential in mitigating the potential centrifugal effects of a heterogeneous, dispersed division of labour so that patients receive timely and integrated care and organisational resources are efficiently utilised. This is important work, which has implications for the care of individual patients and also the efficiency of the organisation, but it is not without its challenges. One of the advantages of shining light on this invisible element of the nursing function is that it reveals some of the barriers that need to be overcome in order for nurses to realise their potential.

Notes

1 At the time of writing, the RCN reported that the NHS has lost nearly 4,000 senior nursing posts since 2010 (www.bbc.co.uk/news/health-26519324, accessed 14 March 2014).
2 Crystallisation point is a term used in actor-network-theory to refer to a summation of a network's activity.

References

Allen, D. (1997). 'The medical-nursing boundary: A negotiated order?' *Sociology of Health & Illness* 19(4): 498–520.
—— (2001). *The Changing Shape of Nursing Practice: The Role of Nurses in the Hospital Division of Labour.* London, Routledge.
—— (2014). 'Lost in translation? "Evidence" and the articulation of institutional logics in integrated care pathways: from positive to negative boundary object.' *Sociology of Health & Illness.* Article first published online 17th March 2014: DOI: 10.1111/1467-95666.12111.
Bardram, J. (2000). 'Temporal coordination. On time and coordination of collaborative activities at a surgical department.' *Computer Supported Cooperative Work* 9: 157–187.
Bardram, J.E. and C. Bossen (2005). 'Mobility work: the spatial dimensions of collaboration at a hospital.' *Computer Supported Cooperative Work* 14: 131–160.
BBC (2012). Secret Scottish NHS incident reports released.
Berg, B. (1992). 'The social construction of medical disposals: medical sociology and medical problem solving in clinical practice.' *Sociology of Health & Illness* 14(2): 151–180.
Bittner, E. (1965). 'The concept of organisation.' *Social Research* 32: 239–255.
Bloor, M. (1976). 'Bishop Berkeley and the adenotonsillectomy enigma: an exploration of variation in the social construction of medical disposals.' *Sociology* 10(1): 43–61.
Bourdieu, P. (2000). *Pascalian Meditations.* Stanford, CA, Stanford University Press.

Cabitza, F., Sarini, M. and C. Simone (2007). Providing awareness through situated process maps: the hospital care case. Group07, Sanibel Island, Florida, USA, ACM.

Callon, M. (1986). Some elements of a sociology of translation: domestication of the scallops and the fishermen of St Brieuc's bay. *Power, Action and Belief. A New Sociology of Knowledge?* J. Law. London, Routledge and Kegan Paul: 196–229.

Clarke, K. and S. Wheelwright (1992). 'Organizing and leading "heavyweight" development teams.' *California Management Review* 34(3): 9–28.

Cohen, M. and P. Bacdayan (1994). 'Organizational routines are stored as procedural memory: evidence from a laboratory study.' *Organizational Science* 5: 554–568.

Davies, C. (1995). *Gender and the Professional Predicament in Nursing.* Buckingham, Open University Press.

DiMaggio, P.J. and W.W. Powell (1983). 'The iron cage revisited: institutional isomorphism and collective rationality in organizational fields.' *American Sociological Review* 48(April): 147–160.

Draycott, T., Sibanda, T., Owen, L., Akande, V., Winter, C., Reading, S. and A. Whitelaw (2006). 'Does training in obstetric emergencies improve neonatal outcome?' *BJOG: an International Journal of Obstetrics and Gynaecology* 113(2): 177–182.

Feldman, M. and B.T. Pentland (2003). 'Reconceptualizing organizational routines as a source of flexibility and change.' *Administrative Science Quarterly* 48: 94–118.

Gittel, J.H., Fairfield, K.M., Bierbaum, B., Head, W., Jackson, R., Kelly, M., Laskin, R., Lipson, S., Siliski, J., Thornhill, T. and Zuckerman, J. (2000). 'Impact of relational coordination on quality of care, postoperative pain and functioning and length of stay.' *Medical Care* 38: 807–819.

Glouberman, S. and H. Mintzberg (2001). 'Managing the care of health and the cure of disease – Part 1: Differentiation.' *Health Care Management Review* Winter: 56–69.

—— (2001). 'Managing the care of health and the cure of disease – part II: integration.' *Health Care Managment Review* 26(1): 70–89.

Goodwin, D. (2013) 'Decision-making and accountability: differences of distribution.' *Sociology of Health & Illness* 36(1): 44–59.

House of Commons (2010). Independent Inquiry into Care Provided by Mid Staffordshire NHS Foundation Trust January 2005 – March 2009, Volumes I and II, (Chaired by Robert Francis QC), HC375. London, The Stationery Office.

—— (2013). Report of the Mid Staffordshire NHS Foundation Trust Public Inquiry, Volumes I, II and III (Chaired by Robert Francis QC), HC 898. London, The Stationery Office.

Latimer, J. (2000). *The Conduct of Care: Understanding Nursing Practice.* Oxford, Blackwells.

Manias, E. and A. Street (2001). 'Nurse-doctor interactions during critical care ward rounds.' *Journal of Clinical Nursing* 10(4): 442–450.

March, J.G. and H. Simon (1958). *Organizations.* New York, Wiley.

Mohr, J.J. and P.B. Batalden (2002). 'Improving safety on the front lines: the role of clinical microsystems.' *Quality & Safety Health Care* 11: 45–50.

National Patient Safety Agency (2007). The Fifth Report from the Patient Safety Observatory. Safer Care for the Acutely Ill Patient: Learning from Serious Incidents. London, National Patient Safety Agency.

Pentland, B.T. and M.S. Feldman (2005). 'Organizational routines as a unit of analysis.' *Industrial and Corporate Change* 14(5): 793–815.

—— (2008). 'Designing routines: on the folly of designing artifacts, while hoping for patterns of action.' *Information and Organization* 18(4): 235–250.

Rapley, T. (2008). 'Distributed decision making: the automony of decisions-in-action.' *Sociology of Health & Illness* 30(3): 429–444.

Salas, E., Rosen, M.A. and H. King (2007). 'Managing teams managing crisis: principles of teamwork to improve patient safety in the emergency room and beyond.' *Theoretical Issues in Ergonomics Science* 8: 381–394.

Silbey, S.S. (2009). 'Taming prometheus: talk about safety and culture.' *Annual Review of Sociology* 35(1): 341–369.

Star, S.L. and A. Strauss (1999). 'Layers of silence, arenas of voice: the ecology of visible and invisible work.' *Computer Supported Cooperative Work* 8: 9–30.

Strauss, A. (1985). 'Work and the division of labor.' *The Sociological Quarterly* 26(1): 1–19.

Strauss, A., Fagerhaugh, S. and B. Suczet (1985). *The Social Organisation of Medical Work*. Chicago, University of Chicago Press.

Telegraph Reporters (2012). Patients die due to flat batteries in hospital equipment. *Telegraph*.

Vygotsky, L. (1978). *Mind in Society: The Development of Higher Psychological Processes*. Cambridge, MA., Harvard University Press.

Waterworth, S. (2003) 'Temporal reference frameworks and nurses' work organization.' *Time and Society* 12(1): 41–54.

Whyte, W.F. (1979). The social structure of the restaurant. *Social Interaction: Introductory Readings in Sociology*. H. Robboy, S.L. Greenblatt and C. Clark. New York, St Martin's Press.

4   Match-making

Patients 'dying' in surgery wait, claims Powys GP (6 September 2013).

A & E doctors say pressure is threat to patient safety (8 October 2013).

Ambulances 'face long delays at A&E – BBC figures reveal (9 December 2013).

Key NHS operations 'being rationed' (6 December 2013).

Broomfield Hospital: Cancer surgery cancelled five times (10 October 2012).
(BBC Health News)

In this chapter I examine the nursing contribution to bed management. 'Beds' are hospitals' primary resource. They are a key feature of the topography of healthcare systems and the currency through which they are organised. The physical and emotional costs to those who cannot access a bed when needed are high, as are the political and financial consequences for organisations and governments when there are queues in emergency departments or operations are cancelled because beds are unavailable. So that simple three letter word – bed – is saturated with meaning and matters a lot. Of course a bed is not just a physical artefact; it includes the associated people, knowledge, space and technology. Hospitals are becoming increasingly specialised and their infrastructures, internal processes and skill-mix are rationally ordered to meet the needs of particular patient populations. As we have seen (Chapter 3), nurses' knowledge of these local activity systems is central to their work in articulating patient trajectories and 'outliers' present certain challenges to their practice. Assigning people to the right bed with all the accompanying resources this confers therefore has important implications for the quality, safety and efficiency of healthcare.

Hospitals face a daily challenge of balancing the demands of an unknown and variable volume of patients and ensuring a sufficient but not excessive number of beds is available for individuals with differing needs (Comptroller and Auditor General 2000). Queuing theory and simulation techniques from operations research readily demonstrate that any production system subject to fluctuations from its environment will cease to perform efficiently if utilisation approaches 100 per cent. The application of these ideas to healthcare has produced a target bed occupancy figure of 85 per cent (Bagust *et al.* 1999). Yet at the time of the study, hospitals in England were operating at a much higher level (90 per cent) (Dr Foster Intelligence 2012) and, according to a senior source, at Parklands this was even higher. When organisations are functioning in such circumstances, patients cannot be placed in the appropriate beds and/or must be moved around the system to create capacity. This makes bed management tremendously challenging. As I have argued, discharge planning processes and care coordination are more demanding for outlying patients and can be disrupted when patients move between wards (Walford 2002). At the time of writing, regular reports in the UK media detailed the growing pressures in emergency units and expanding waiting lists for elective surgery as a result of increased attendances and insufficient bed capacity.

Optimising acute bed-utilisation by the proactive management of patient journeys through the service was a priority at Parklands and during the period of my observations, the pressure on beds was immense. Those with a long familiarity with the organisation observed that each year the intensity of bed-utilisation had grown and what were once seasonal pressures had become a steady state. Two contrasting logics of bed-utilisation were in circulation. On the one hand, a logic of efficiency underlined the importance of allocating acute beds to those categories of patient that could benefit most from them.

> Specialist Nurse: 'It isn't acceptable any longer to say to a patient that they can stay a couple more days when you have others in the corridors in Accident and Emergency and Day Surgery taking the overflow.'

On the other hand, a logic of individualised care highlighted how maximising bed-utilisation overshadowed the needs of specific patients. This is captured in the following extract in which a senior nurse evokes the image of hospital bureaucrats applying abstract impersonal rules to allocate beds.

> They wanted us to allocate the dependency levels on the white board so that the clip board carriers could come and see who was level 2 and who was level 3. They don't know what they mean but they had some rule.

These positions were not aligned with particular groups or individuals. Indeed, I heard both logics evoked by the same people in different contexts. They are not about world views, but might better be understood as indicative of the tensions – the conflicting institutional logics – that bisected the organisation as it endeavoured to reconcile the needs of individuals with the needs of the many. I have no doubt that everyone who worked at Parklands felt these pressures. But nurses felt them particularly acutely.

Beds: a nursing responsibility

Historically in the UK, acute sector beds were managed at ward level, but over the last 30 years, as demand has grown, the hospital has emerged as the main functional unit (Green and Armstrong 1993). The period has also witnessed a shift in control away from consultants to nurses employed in formal bed management roles. In line with UK national guidance (Comptroller and Auditor General 2000), at Parklands, the patient access and discharge liaison nurses had primary responsibility for bed-utilisation. Nevertheless, beyond these specialist roles, nurses throughout the organisation, from ward to board, were enrolled in bed management.

At ward level, all patients were required to have a planned discharge date and achieving this was a key performance indicator for unit managers. Ward nurses were thus oriented both to the patients in their immediate care and those that might benefit from it in the future. Activities related to discharge planning were prioritised with staff working hard to ensure these took place before midday and, once vacated, beds were instantly available. Indeed it was these pressures that had provided the impetus for the development of the coordinator role. Beyond the patient care areas, anaesthetic pre-assessment nurses evaluated individuals' fitness for surgery to avoid cancelled operations after admission and many other specialist roles included a bed management component. Thus the stroke coordinator aimed to ensure that patients were 'in the right place [...] as soon as possible where there is more experience in the way of therapy [...] and then move[d] on in 7 days'; the cardiology coordinator, determined whether referrals were 'hot, or have cooled down and [could] wait a couple of days', and the rehabilitation nurse specialist looked 'at the referrals or in fact [went to] find them and assess their suitability for rehabilitation on behalf of the consultant'. Furthermore, in addition to the patient access nurses, in other parts of the organisation nurses worked in roles exclusively concerned with bed management. The Emergency Unit coordinator mobilised patient pathways through the department, the Medical and Surgical Assessment Unit coordinators interceded between the Emergency Unit and the wards, and the site manager assumed responsibility for bed allocation outside core hours.

In the upper organisational echelons, senior nurses met weekly to bring their skills to bear on cases categorised as delayed transfers of care (those patients considered medically fit but who remained in hospital). They also supervised the quality of applications for continuing healthcare, so these did not invite opposition from the funding panel and delay discharge. I learnt, too, that plans were in place for student nurses to have clinical placements with the patient access nurses and it was becoming increasingly common for newly-appointed nurses to spend time with the team so they might better understand the pressures under which they worked. Nurses throughout the organisation were thus comprehensively enrolled in the bed management agenda. Through a number of gate-keeping roles, nurses determined on any given day who had access to the service; expediting timely discharges was almost exclusively a nursing responsibility; and allocating patients to the appropriate bed, once an administrative function, was now the work of nurses.

Match-making

In various ways across a multitude of roles, nurses at Parklands were engaged in allocating beds and overseeing the movement of patients through the system. When beds are plentiful, this is not unduly challenging work; indeed historically it has been undertaken by administrative staff. In conditions of intense demand, however, bed management requires skilled judgement in order to meet the needs of individuals while maximising bed-utilisation. This entailed an iterative process of moving from one possible coupling to another in order to bring about the necessary translations to accomplish optimal arrangements. I have used the notion of match-making to capture this work.[1] At Parklands, match-making placed different demands on nurses at different points in the system, but a common thread was the requirement for the synthesis of clinical and organisational knowledge.

What is a bed?

What is a bed? This is a simple question for which there is a complex answer. Even if we limit our discussion to material artefacts, we discover a wide variety: hospital beds, paediatric beds, bariatric beds, low-rise beds. Trolleys too may be used as beds, but only for certain kinds of patient and for a limited period. The word is also associated with different kinds of expertise and equipment. There are intensive care beds, cardiology beds, an array of surgical beds, and never enough medical beds. There is a range of rehabilitation beds: fast track, slow stream and subtle gradations in between. There are beds reserved for short-term use, such as the 'bed and breakfast' beds in Intensive Care and the 'bed and board' beds in the Short Stay Surgical Unit. Outside the acute sector there are nursing home beds, residential home beds, transitional care beds, and continuing health care beds. There are beds for the elderly mentally infirm and dual registered beds for patients with mental and physical health needs. Of course people have their own beds in their homes, but may need additional support and attachments to safely sleep in them.

Beds are not just associated with expertise but also staff. Without sufficient staff, operations cannot take place or wards reach the limits of their capacity to care. Even within the same department, not all beds are equal. Certain beds are in spaces that make them more-or-less suited to particular kinds of patient. In the Medical Assessment Unit, additional beds had been created to increase capacity, but they were not clearly visible and therefore could only be used for 'low-risk patients'. Throughout the organisation, a premium was placed on 'cubicles', that is, beds in a single room, because these could be used flexibly for men or women, whereas the organisation's commitment to same sex accommodation meant that those in the main ward areas could not (although intensive care units and theatre recovery were the exception to this rule). Cubicles were also required for patients at risk of infection. Parklands, like other hospitals, had a pool of beds that could be accessed flexibly to create extra capacity. The Short Stay Surgical Unit was used regularly to cope with pressures in the system, but was only able to accommodate patients of particular kinds.

> Coordinator: 'We can't safely look after very sick patients, the unit is too busy with our normal work and we're too removed from the rest of the hospital, so they are not in a good place.'

In all likelihood I have missed other important distinctions, but the point is that 'beds' are a complex currency which nurses were required to understand in order to find the right fit for patient need.

What is a patient?

Alongside their nuanced understanding of beds, nurses worked with a parallel schema of patients. It is well-recognised that health professionals typify patients according to their medical condition. Referring to someone as 'the appendicectomy in bed 6' is criticised for its dehumanising effects, but nonetheless it still happens. It still happens, because as I have argued, human subjects do not relate to the objective world directly; activity is always mediated by artefacts. In this context, categories of patient, just as categories of bed, are psychological artefacts (Vygotsky 1978) and useful for the purposes of organising everyday service delivery. Indeed, the study of such artefacts may tell us something about the nature of this work. When we shine a light on nurses' bed management what emerges is a professional vision[2] (Goodwin 1994) based on categories of patient that related in part to their medical condition but, more accurately, to their relevance for the allocation of beds in the particular local economies for which nurses were responsible. For example, the classifications deployed by the Emergency Unit coordinators reflected the need to place patients in the topography of beds available in their immediate areas. They made reference to 'jumpers' (patients at risk of falls by climbing out of bed) and CIWA[3] patients (patients undergoing withdrawal from alcohol and who were known to become agitated) both of whom were required to be placed in high visibility beds.

> Coordinator asks whether the patient's comprehension is OK.
>
> Staff Nurse says that it is fine and 'she doesn't seem to be a jumper'.
>
> We go to the Medical Assessment Unit.

Staff Nurse: '8 is free. I can take the CIWA.'

Coordinator explained that these patients 'need to be visible because they were quite disruptive. They are likely to climb off the trolley'.

Medical beds were under immense pressure, and although the Medical Assessment Unit was the first choice for allocating patients after they had been seen in the Emergency Unit, it was sometimes necessary to use the Surgical Assessment Unit beds in order to manage flows. But not all medical patients were appropriate for such placement and Emergency Unit staff had an eye for those individuals who might be suitable for transfer. Similarly, on the Medical Assessment Unit, the nurses were attuned to those patients fit enough to be moved to the wards on trolleys as was sometimes necessary when the pressures in the system increased, and in the Surgical Assessment Unit, as well as assigning patients to the appropriate service categories, the nurses also routinely identified those patients who could be transferred to the Short Stay Surgical Unit if it was being used as additional bed capacity. It was rarely necessary to specify the exact features that rendered patients an appropriate match, this was part of the taken-for-granted knowledge of unit staff and the work of managing patient flows depended on summative assessments of patients who were categorised according to the bed types in which they could be placed.

On the wards, nurses drew on a range of patient types in discussions about bed allocation, but it was in decisions around transfers of care that patient categorisation as a constituent of the match-making process was most evident. Again, categories of patient were understood in terms of their match with a particular service.

Physiotherapist: 'She sat out of bed today but she's very weak. She might be FRAME.' ((Functional Rehabilitation and Medical Evaluation bed))

Discharge Liaison Nurse: 'Is she FRAME?'

Rehabilitation Nurse: 'Sounds more like FRAME.'

Discharge Liaison Nurse: 'He's got slow stream rehabilitation written all over him.'

From an outside position, such categorisation processes make healthcare look like a production line. It sounds bad and uncaring. People – you, me, mothers, fathers, children – disappear from view. Yet these are very effective mechanisms for condensing large amounts of organisationally relevant information into a form that enables decision-making. This was a necessary effacement of individual identities in order to understand the relationships between patients and beds necessary to accomplish the work. Indeed, so close was the coupling of patient categories with beds that in some instances staff were able to infer patient details from the bed-type that was requested.

Rehabilitation Nurse calls the ward: 'Can I give you a name for a male bed? [] he's on Snowdrop Ward. He needs a low-rise bed mind.'

[...] A few minutes later Rehabilitation Nurse is bleeped.

Rehabilitation Nurse ((To me)): 'That will be the ward saying there are no low-rise beds.'

She proves to be right. The ward already has three patients on low-rise beds and the dependency levels on the ward are such that they cannot take anyone else.

Rehabilitation Nurse: 'They are quite good. If they say they can't take him they can't. Have you been to Spring Rehabilitation Ward? It was built in the 1960s according to Victorian standards and was originally a maternity hospital. You can't see people on the unit and they have 40 patients on there with minimal staffing. They know if I ask for a low-rise bed there might be issues.'

When the rehabilitation nurse requests a low-rise bed, the ward nurse is able to gauge the proposed admission's dependency level on the basis of the bed-type required. Low-rise beds typically are used for patients at risk of falls, which in this setting more often than not is owing to cognitive impairment. Such patients require high levels of care. Signalling very clearly the relationship between beds and resources, the ward indicates that while there are 'beds' available, currently they have inadequate staff capacity to care for such a dependent patient. And, as my respondent summarises in terms that powerfully reveal the close coupling of patient identities with beds: 'they have three low-rise beds and they won't manage another.'

Having an overview of capacity and demand

Nurses were expected to have an overview of bed availability in their areas and this required them to draw on their fine-grained understanding of the local bed currency and their knowledge of patients, to assess and review capacity. At the front door of the hospital, the coordinators worked to keep the Emergency Unit operational, and this meant ensuring it had empty beds. Key areas of concern were the Medical and Surgical Assessment Units where patients were moved once they had been seen by EU doctors and referred to the relevant clinical teams. Throughout the shift, the coordinator visited these areas over and over again to maintain oversight of bed capacity and patient flows into the main hospital wards. In turn the coordinators in each unit worked continuously to retain an overview of the bed situation in their respective areas. As we saw in the previous chapter, white boards were an important tool through which they carried out this work. In order to appraise demand, nurses had also to anticipate patients most likely to require beds. In the Medical Assessment Unit, the coordinators reviewed the brief clinical details on the GP referral list to assess patients likely to need admission. Nurses quickly identified the 'barn door' patients, that is, those whose pattern of signs and symptoms pointed to a well-known clinical condition and trajectory pathway. Although responsibility for requesting admission ultimately resided with medical staff, the ability to read from the brief clinical details available and anticipate likely demand was an important skill that enabled coordinators to plan ahead.

> In the Trolley Bay area Coordinator asks whether 'any are likely to be passing trade' but the nurse says that most are likely to be admitted.

The Short Stay Surgical Unit was another critical node in the overall system and bed management in this context was particularly complex. The unit was frequently used as additional capacity for the rest of the organisation and, as a consequence, the ward coordinators were required to engage in complex processes of predicting the trajectories of patients in order to identify bed availability so that they could make judgements about whether surgical lists would be able to go ahead. They also operated with a mixture of beds and trolleys which could be used flexibly, but which were more-or-less suitable for certain patients dependent on age and the nature of their surgery. Caught between the dual pressures of scheduled and unscheduled care, I observed the coordinators engaged in careful work to assess the likely movement of patients through the service and how beds might be used to maximum capacity. In the following extract the coordinator and service manager review bed availability and assess its implications for which theatre cases can take place.

> Coordinator: 'At the moment we have got two males and two trolleys by the looks of it.' (('Males' actually refers to beds rather than people)).
>
> Senior Manager: 'We haven't got a female?'
>
> Coordinator: 'There's three trolleys so the female could go on the trolley. What is it?'
>
> Senior Manager: 'Cystoscopy.'
>
> Coordinator: 'That's fine as long as it goes home and doesn't bleed.'
>
> Senior manager checks the date of birth of the patient. She is 80 and both Coordinator and Senior manager are concerned about putting an 80 year old on a trolley. They resume looking at the board.
>
> Senior Manager: 'What about []?'
>
> Coordinator: 'He's a pain.' ((Someone on the pain theatre list)).
>
> Senior Manager: '[Male patient's name currently in one of two cubicles] could be a female.'

Coordinator: 'OK so that's three males, one cube and say four trolleys possibly.'

Senior Manager ((Points to board)): 'What about this lot?'

Coordinator: 'No they're two [name of consultant] and an ERCP ((Endoscopic Retrograde Cholangiopancreatography)) so they'll be staying.'

Beyond the work involved in managing beds in these local economies, it was the patient access nurses who were charged with maintaining an overview of the shape of the organisation as a whole. At the time of the study, Parklands did not have a computerised integrated bed management system, although one was under development. Information on predicted discharge dates was available centrally but widely recognised to be inaccurate. Nurses struggled to find the time to update the database and, because the central system was used to monitor ward performance on discharge planning, there was an element of disconnection between the actual mechanisms of discharge management and the work involved in managing the presentation of data relating to these processes. As a consequence, the patient access nurses expended considerable time and energy clarifying and collating information to maintain as accurate a picture as possible of the bed state in their areas of responsibility. This entailed visiting the wards and holding conversations with the nurse in charge. Previous studies have suggested that it is necessary for bed managers to visit wards in order to uncover gaming, such as beds being hidden or not declared by staff in order to manage their work. But this was not regarded as a major issue at Parklands. While I witnessed one example of a bed remaining empty over night, this was widely assumed to be an error, rather than a deliberate attempt to mislead. In addition to the ward visits, the Patient Access Team held meetings three times a day in order to review beds which included senior nurses from key areas and directorate managers. When bed pressures were particularly acute, these meetings had the flavour of a war cabinet and, as well as providing an overview of the bed state, appeared to function to generate a state of collective purpose. In the following extract derived from the morning meeting, the senior nurse reports on a difficult night. There are patients in the corridor in the Emergency Unit and GP referrals have been redirected to another hospital in order to ease the pressure. The reference to the rehabilitation nurse in this extract points to her role in moving patients from acute wards into rehabilitation beds in order to create capacity. Here we can see that bed management is as much about matching patients to suitable beds as it is about finding patients who can be allocated to empty beds elsewhere in the system to allow flows into the hospital.

Senior Nurse: 'It's been a very difficult night. There have been patients in the corridor most of the night, and there were 11 at one point. The GP intake is going to Valley Hospital and it sounds as if Valley Hospital has beds. Rehabilitation Nurse is not here but they have empty beds and

I will email her afterwards. There are some long waits on trolleys. We need to prioritise as they are all on trolleys.'

At the different sites of the healthcare system, then, nurses were engaged in assigning patients to beds. This entailed a process of match-making in which clinical and organisational knowledge was synthesised to bring about a fit between patient needs and available resources. It took place in a difficult context in which nurses were caught up in the tensions of balancing the needs of individuals with the needs of the many. In the second half of this chapter I will offer some examples of match-making in action, highlighting along the way the skills and knowledge this work reveals.

Match-making in action

Patient access nurses and site managers

Patient access nurses and the out-of-hours site managers were responsible for maximising overall bed-utilisation at Parklands and making a good match between beds requested and those available. These negotiations could be challenging. If a bed could not be located in the service under which the patient was to be admitted, then compromises had to be reached, things had to be 'jiggled around' and the next best fit found. In order to secure such accommodations, finely-tuned clinical skills and a sophisticated understanding of the organisational topography of beds was necessary in which the needs of the patient requiring a bed had to be balanced with those of the other patients cared for in a service.

> Patient Access Nurse said that for the purposes of placing people in a suitable bed wider clinical information was necessary. She gave the example of chest pain. 'Chest pain can be a chest infection, PE ((pulmonary embolism)), cardiac, it can be someone who has a spinal injury. It's important to know this wider information.'
>
> Site Manager: 'Sometimes there are a number of patients in the system that need beds and you may have to look at the notes and see what is suitable for an outlier if we need to move them into beds and off of trolleys.'

These were also political decisions. Owing to a combination of risk and performance management concerns, today's health providers operate with a circumscribed view of service shape (Strauss *et al.* 1985) and individual units are designed around a particular kind of client and/or processes. Yet despite this increased rationalisation and specialisation, at Parklands it was necessary for beds to be used flexibly to accommodate system pressures. Thus at any one time, most wards would have a number of 'outliers' where the responsible clinical team was ordinarily associated with another ward. While outliers create challenges for medical staffs because the patients under their care are widely dispersed across the organisation, they do not impact on the content of their work, whereas they had a marked effect on that of nurses. As I have shown, the needs of such patients could extend nurses beyond their normal areas of expertise and also create problems for trajectory coordination owing to their unfamiliarity with network actors. It was also the case that in certain units the physical environment and organisational infrastructure was not able to accommodate easily patients of particular kinds. Nurses throughout the organisation were engaged in a continuous process of managing the shape of their own services. Patient access nurses and site managers functioned with an acute sensitivity to these concerns and, in allocating patients to outlying areas, took care not to over extend the goodwill of unit staff by as far as possible assigning cases whose needs closely resembled the patients team members were accustomed to caring for.

> Site Manager: 'When the neuro wards have got beds and the flows are bad we will use them. We try and keep it vaguely neuro say CVA (stroke) and try to keep to the sort of speciality.'

There were particular sensitivities about placing confused patients, primarily because they were known to be demanding and there was relatively little capacity on the wards to cope with patients of this kind.

> Site Manager: 'If you are trying to place someone on CIWA you can't find a bed anywhere. I wouldn't out-lie such patients as they can be disruptive.'

> Patient Access Nurse (Surgery): 'Any cubicle required?'

> Patient Access Nurse (Medicine): 'One of my confused patients!!!'

> Patient Access Nurse (Surgery): 'Oh no! You can't do that!!'

Effecting transfers of care entailed subtle negotiations in order to place patients. Sometimes this entailed returning one of the unit's 'own' patients from an outlying area as part of a deal struck to accept a new admission. We might think of this as 'trading patients' which, rather like the work of 'selling patients' (Nugus *et al.* 2009), is a further mechanism by which patients are moved along and placed within the system. I saw lots of these sorts of compromises and it was through such negotiations and bargaining that the organisation continued to function. Nevertheless, it is undeniable that difficult compromises were sometimes necessary.

> Patient Access Nurse observes: 'It's not bad but they are not where you would want them.'

When pressures were really intense additional beds had to be created. This entailed making politically charged decisions about using the Short Stay

Surgical Unit to increase capacity. There was considerable sensitivity about how these beds were utilised, and there was widespread sympathy about the impact this had on staff.

> Coordinator said that the volume of outlying patients on the unit was a source of stress for staff. 'They would rather look after their own than the outliers. They know these come with baggage and issues and they have not signed up for that. [...] Sometimes the patients are very rude and the relatives are very rude and when they find out they are in the wrong place they think that they are not being looked after.'

There were other costs: extra staff had to be booked and families notified about cancelled operations. When all such efforts failed, senior nurses were forced to prioritise scheduled admissions, typically patients with a cancer diagnosis. There was no evidence of special pleading or 'shroud waving',[4] however; all worked with a shared sense of justness, echoing Green and Armstrong's (1995) observations about the rhetoric of neutrality in the rational allocation of beds that has emerged with bed management.

The work of the patient access nurses required them to shift backwards and forwards between a clinical and an organisational gaze and to zoom in and out, moving between their understanding of the overall hospital bed state and their assessment of the needs of particular individuals. They did this work in immensely pressurised circumstances, in a rapidly changing but often uncertain and contingent organisational scene. They also operated with an acute sensitivity to the needs of ward-based staff to control the shape of their units.

Unscheduled care

While the Patient Access Team was responsible for finding and allocating beds, elsewhere nurses made decisions about bed allocation before patients were admitted. In bringing the individual into the organisation, the Emergency Unit triage nurse was required to consider where to place patients. Such judgements were taken against the backdrop of high demand and the requirement to ensure beds were available at all times. Match-making in this context might entail not allocating a 'bed' if the patient could be cared for elsewhere.

> Triage Nurse explained that if she had patients who were unlikely to be admitted she tends not to put them into a cubicle so that they don't take up a space in the department.

Whereas the patient access nurses' work entailed deliberative processes of zooming in and zooming out, trading patients and planning ahead for contingencies, allocating beds at the front door of the service required rapid assessment and decision-making. In the following extract, the Emergency Unit coordinator intervenes to clear a backlog while the triage nurse is attending to another patient.

> Whilst Triage Nurse is with the patient who has complained, Coordinator triages the other patients waiting with the crews. One lady has been fallen on by another resident in a residential home and cut her arm; the paramedic is directed to take her to the Triage Room in her wheelchair. A man, on a trolley, has had a fainting episode in the pub and is moved further down the corridor to await a bed with Coordinator saying that she is happy to go with the paramedic's observations. The third lady was shopping and experienced pain in her arm and jaw; she took her GTN ((Glyceryl Trinitrate)) and then got to Superdrug 'as they are nice to her in there' where she vomited and is continuing to experience pain. Coordinator directs her straight into 'Resus' and asks them to do a '12 lead' ((ECG)). A young woman has hurt her ankle playing rugby. It is splinted and Coordinator assesses it. It is clearly painful. She redirects her to Minors.[5] Having cleared the backlog in a remarkably short period of time, Coordinator then hands over to Triage Nurse.

Sometimes placing patients in difficult circumstances meant making compromises.

> As we return to the corridor we greet a paramedic dealing with an aggressive male patient. He has learning disabilities and is postictal. He is shouting and lashing out at the paramedics who describe him as 'very combative'. One of the team is calmly speaking to him telling him to 'relax'. Another patient arrives at the entrance and Triage Nurse asks the paramedics to move the patient straight into the cubicle.
>
> Staff Nurse asks: 'Is he safe to be left in there on his own?'
>
> Triage Nurse: 'What choice have I got? The corridor?'

Some patients were clearly considered more deserving of a space than others. For example, during one set of field observations I noticed that for most of the shift two 'regulars' were left in the corridor on trolleys to sleep off the effects of alcohol after which they would be discharged. In contrast, a bed was quickly found for a lady who presented at the department, bleeding from recent haemorrhoidectomy surgery. That emergency unit staffs operate with such notions of social justice is well-recognised (Jeffery 1979; Dingwall and Murray 1983; Vassy 2001; Hillman 2013).

Beyond the front door pressures, the coordinator worked to move patients out of the department into the Medical and Surgical Assessment Units, liaising continuously to establish which beds were available and who could be assigned to them. In the following extract, the coordinator has identified a space in the Medical Assessment Unit and is trying to fill it to release the bed in the Emergency Unit. When the doctor volunteers a patient, notice how the coordinator reads from the clinical information provided and translates this into the type of bed that will be required ('so it will need monitoring') which limits the kind of space they can occupy in the unit.

> Standing in the middle of the High Dependency Unit office Coordinator says, 'I need a medical patient who can go to Medical Assessment Unit'. One of the doctors says that he might have one, 'Tachycardia, no precipitating factors'.
>
> Coordinator: 'So it will need ((cardiac)) monitoring.'

As this example reveals, in the Emergency Unit managing throughput was often focused less on finding beds for patients as it was identifying patients who could be moved into the available beds in order to 'maintain flow'.

On the wards

The match-making metaphor works too for the processes involved in effecting transfers of care at ward level which, given the pressures on beds, always took place in conditions of time and resource constraint. Acute services are obliged to discharge patients when they can no longer benefit from them and yet rehabilitation and community services are hugely stretched. Thus in expediting patient flows, nurses operated with a degree of clinical pragmatism in which they endeavoured to reconcile the needs of individuals with the organisational imperative to expedite a timely discharge. This is encapsulated in the following field note in which a ward coordinator is expressing frustration with a consultant's insistence on a singular discharge destination in the context of a bed being unavailable when the nurses' preference is to negotiate alternative arrangements.

> Coordinator: 'We had a big argument about the lady in there yesterday [...]. Consultant wants her to go to Transitional Care Unit but they are chocker and so we've been doing an alternative safe discharge plan. Her overall goal is for home but he's like "No no she's for Transitional Care Unit because if she likes it there she can stay". I know we should be giving her every option but she's blocking an acute hospital bed and if we leave her here she's just going to end up with an infection. [...] Anyway Discharge Liaison Nurse got stuck into him. [...] He has a patient focus – and insists that she needs a Transitional Care Unit bed and that's fine but they are not moving. We live in the real world where we can't have this lady in an acute bed when we have patients in the corridor in A&E and outliers on surgical wards so we have to look for alternatives. He's thinking about the patient, we're thinking about the whole system.'

This extract is interesting for what it reveals about the articulation of the different logics in play within the organisation, expressed by the coordinator as the contrast between the 'patient focus' of the consultant and 'the real world' inhabited by the nurses. The point is that navigating these tensions in order to agree a discharge from hospital entailed artful processes in order to secure a fit between the individual and the available services. In the following example, the team discuss the needs of a patient they anticipate will soon be ready for discharge. Their preference is to refer her to Stellar, a community-based rehabilitation team designed to 'help people get back up to speed' after a period of illness, or the onset of a disability, but this will create a delay in her discharge home. So they elect to arrange for an alternative service, which is less well-suited to her needs, but quicker to put in place.

Social Worker: 'Can we refer her to Stellar?'

Occupational Therapist: 'They've changed their policy; you can't make a referral until she is ready to go.'

Social Worker: 'But then there will be a delay.'

Occupational Therapist: 'There's no point in referring her now, it will just bounce back.'

Consultant: 'Does she need Stellar?'

Occupational Therapist: 'Yes she needs assistance to mobilise.'

Coordinator: 'The trouble is it's Thursday now.'

Consultant: 'The other option is that she went with Quantum but that would mean she would not have physio for next week.'

Social Worker: 'It's a big gap.'

SHO: 'Next week? It's unfortunate isn't it?'

Coordinator: 'How long does it take?'

Occupational Therapist: 'Stellar the last time it has taken a couple of weeks, they have no capacity to even screen.'

Consultant: 'That's a non-starter.'

Occupational Therapist: 'Yeah, we'll probably have to go down the Quantum route.'

Equally, however, operating in circumstances of resource constraint, many community-based services had referral criteria in order to control their workload. In such circumstances, negotiating a match entailed 'making a case' for a particular level of provision. At Parklands a unified assessment form was used for these purposes. However, although purportedly an objective assessment of need, the documentation was used to fabricate patient identities in order to ensure that the 'assessed needs' aligned with the requirements of the service and the referral accepted.

> Coordinator: 'The social worker wants Quantum ((community based rehabilitation service)) to go in there and they need the documents to show that they require it. In all honesty you make the document fit the needs of the patient. You know they want Quantum so you make sure you can show that they need it.'

This extract is interesting because while the nurse in question readily acknowledges that there is a political construction at work here, their account appears to orient to a belief in an objective patient identity existing independently of the organisational purposes to which it is being put. As I will argue in Chapter 5, it may be necessary to rethink these assumptions.

Sometimes these careful constructions can create their own problems and new negotiations are required. In the following extract, the discharge liaison nurse negotiates with a nursing home that has refused to accept a patient on the grounds that the only available room cannot accommodate a hoist.

> One nursing home has refused to accept the patient even though they have a room. The room is small and cannot accommodate a hoist. However, Discharge Liaison Nurse argues that the patient will not use a hoist as he does not get out of bed. She says she will contact the home and see if she can 'charm them' and get him accepted into this room until a more suitable one becomes available. 'This chap never wants to get out of bed and will never need a hoist; he knows his own mind. I am going to speak to them. I know him and I'll see if I can sell the picture.'

It was also the case, however, that referral criteria were not always clear to secondary sector staff which could make fabricating identities in order to secure a match more challenging.

> Coordinator said that the other issue they faced was that the residential homes did not have consistent criteria about the kind of patient they were happy to accept. Some would take patients with incontinence, others would not. This makes it very difficult for staff working in the acute sector to identify suitable placements. There was also a view that the criteria were deliberately kept vague so that residential homes could 'cherry pick' the patients they liked and refuse those they did not.

While the reference to cherry picking in this extract is not without some foundation, ambiguous referral criteria allow organisations flexibility to control access to beds based on an overall assessment of capacity. As we saw in the earlier example of the low-rise bed, it is possible for 'beds' to be available, but not the other associated actors necessary to ensure quality of care. Nevertheless, match-making was clearly confounded by financial considerations. In Wales, whereas continuing health care is funded by the NHS which is free to all, social care is funded by the local authority and, beyond a certain threshold, is means-tested. Parklands was a regional centre for spinal injuries and the neurological discharge liaison nurse described in great detail the challenges she faced in securing agreements for ongoing care arrangements for her patients, many of whom were eligible for NHS funding. Staff worked hard to organise for a home discharge where possible, but since this group has complex needs, the packages of care were expensive. Furthermore, because patients were often young, providers were concerned about the longer-term financial implications of their care arrangements. She described how negotiating with health authorities was enormously challenging and that making a match required extraordinary amounts of documentation to build the case.

> Discharge Liaison Nurse: 'The panel came back and requested a few more alternative sets of arrangements to a home discharge and information on the risks associated with the home discharge and how we were going to manage them. I was very frustrated since it was clear in the covering letter that the patient's preference was to go home but that there were risks associated with a home discharge. I spoke to the team and said "We have done the risk assessment, the environment is safe", but they said that they wanted us to think about the totality of the care and what would happen if he became ill. I think it took me about a day to pull all that together. It was all in the original care plan but he had not been formally risk assessed.'

Having dealt with repeated challenges to the information on the unified assessment form, she had developed an elaborate formal risk assessment proforma to make transparent the assessments embedded in the recommendations for care in order to marshal stronger evidence for the match being proposed.

> Discharge Liaison Nurse: 'It is very time consuming. It generates a score and you have a revised risk score when a care management plan is in place. It isn't required for all patients; they are not all coming back and asking for evidence. I will do one for the man on Ward 4 as concerns have been raised about his discharge destination.'

Beyond the growing work of fabricating a case for a package of care through a range of formal artefacts, the discharge liaison nurses, like other nurses, drew on their social capital to facilitate such negotiations. In the following example, the neurological discharge liaison nurse, acting as the patient representative, described a case in which she had used her contacts with a senior nurse to negotiate a transfer when the match in question was being resisted by the Health Board who questioned whether the patient met the Continuing Healthcare Criteria.

> Discharge Liaison Nurse: 'A representative came down from his area to get an overview of his needs. It was a very costly package and there were considerations about the sustainability which are linked into the care planning policy and join into the continuing health care eligibility around whether a care plan is sustainable and not too costly. However they will make exceptions! I met with the senior nurse in the locality. I know her. Over the years you build up a network and an element of trust. I met with her and said he was going back but that they did not want to accept my recommendations. She asked me to explain the rationale to her and why he met the Continuing Healthcare Criteria and she agreed. She trusted my judgement.

In this case, then, the discharge liaison nurse and her senior nurse contact form an alliance in order to represent the interests of the patient in the presentation to the Health Board.

Match-making at the secondary–community interface also entailed negotiations with patients and family members about what was possible. Many of my respondents observed that families had 'unrealistic expectations' of the services that could be provided in the community. An important element of the discharge liaison nurse's role was to manage these expectations in order to reach agreement on suitable discharge destination.

> She said that some families have completely unrealistic expectations of what can be provided in the community for support and that the discharge liaison nurses are helpful in managing these expectations.

Whereas the work of the patient access nurses and unscheduled care staff was concerned with finding beds in order to bring people into the organisation, match-making at ward level was driven by the organisational imperative to move patients out of the hospital once they were considered no longer able to benefit from acute care. In a context of scarce resources this could involve some artful compromises in finding a good enough match in order to avoid delayed discharges and careful negotiations whereby the needs of individuals had to be balanced with that of populations so as to ensure service standards.

Challenges

As these descriptions make clear, match-making took place in time-pressured environments under conditions of resource constraint. Not surprisingly this created tensions. The Emergency Unit coordinators were accused of pushing too hard to empty the department, patient access nurses were labelled as only being interested in finding beds, and ward nurses were charged with organising discharges before patients had been adequately assessed. Indeed, bed management was the primary source of organisational difficulty observed during the fieldwork. I observed instances in which patients admitted for surgery via the Theatre Admissions Lounge[6] were taken to theatre before confirmation that a bed was available on the ward; it was not uncommon for patients to arrive on wards before the bed was ready and there were several cases in which individual's needs were allegedly misrepresented to secure a match leaving the receiving ward ill-equipped to provide their care.

There were also examples of doctors making autonomous decisions about accepting patients without taking into account the organisational consequences. I observed instances of consultants adding cases to the short stay surgical theatre lists without any consideration for whether the unit would have beds available in the post-operative period and last minute clinical decisions about patients' care that had major implications for nursing staff. In one example, a patient was returned to a ward following surgery when it had been intended that they would be monitored in the Intensive Care Unit overnight. The anaesthetist had decided that the patient did not require an intensive care bed. In many ways this was a rational use of a scarce resource, but because it was unplanned there was an inadequate skill-mix on the ward to cope with such a dependent patient and it was too late to organise bank or agency cover. I observed a rather unedifying spectacle as the ward nurse argued with the theatre recovery nurse about whether the patient could be accepted or not, all within earshot of the patient who was parked on his bed in the ward corridor.

As I have argued, pressure on the system required the allocation of beds to be adjusted to generate capacity in those areas where it was needed which meant nurses often sought to identify patients to fill the available beds rather than the other way round. Recent reports on hospital care have highlighted the unacceptability of frequent movement of patients, who are made to feel pushed about and uncared for (House of Commons 2010a, b; Keogh 2013). Officially there was a restriction on the number of times a patient could be moved unless it was for clinical reasons, but these were not too difficult to find and it did appear that patients were moved frequently and often with little notice. I observed numerous occasions in which hospital staffs and family members arrived on ward areas to see individuals who had been transferred to another unit.

Occupational Therapist: '[patient's name]?'

Receptionist: 'She's not here; she's gone to City Hospital.'

Occupational Therapist: 'Oh for goodness sake. I've gone to six patients today and they've not been there. Here's my list and I haven't seen one yet.'

The literature on bed management points to the importance of those charged with this function having authority and legitimacy and a nursing background is widely regarded as affording such credibility (Baillie *et al.* 1997). Yet, previous research has pointed to nurses' ambivalence towards colleagues employed in bed management roles (Green and Armstrong 1993). Green and Armstrong (1993) suggest that nurses' primary attachment is to the ward, whereas doctors and managers orient to the whole organisation and thus as an occupational group, nurses may experience loss of local control over beds more keenly. My data do not lend support for this interpretation, but it is certainly the case that it is the content of nurses' work that is affected most by bed allocation decisions. Green and Armstrong also suggest that against the backcloth of nursing's struggle for professional status, those who undertake bed management roles might be viewed as having 'gone over to the other side'. While I did not observe any overt evidence of conflict, it was clear that the patient access nurses at Parklands occupied an ambiguous position within the organisation. Nurses were particularly critical of the role with a number claiming their clinical skills were largely redundant.

> Nurse: 'Patient Access don't care if we have a patient moved and then they have to be moved back because as long as they are in the system it looks as if they have had a bed.'

> She ((nurse)) said that she understood that it was not an easy job but she didn't think it used any nursing skills simply because there was never any choice about which beds could be used.

Many others, however, expressed sympathy for the patient access nurses and the challenges they faced.

> Senior nurse said the Patient Access Team was subject to terrible abuse from doctors. He said that one was asked for her name by a doctor who had said he needed it 'so that when this patient dies because you couldn't find them a bed I know who to blame'.

> Coordinator said that she has been a deputy ward sister for three months and for part of her induction she spent some time with 'Patient Access'. She said that she found the experience really interesting and it had opened her eyes to the pressures on beds within the hospital. 'We only see issues from our point of view and OK the ward might be busy but there is the wider picture.'

Nurses throughout the organisation were confronted on a daily basis with the need to balance their professional responsibilities for individual patients' quality of care with the needs of whole populations and as we have seen, responsibility for bed management was distributed across the profession. One possible explanation for the ambiguous position of the patient access nurses is that they were a visible embodiment of the tensions inherent in this work.

Despite the importance of their match-making function and the associated clinical and organisational intelligence that informed this work, nurses were largely excluded from strategy making. Shortly before I started my fieldwork, a management decision had been taken to close a 38-bedded medical ward in the belief that more services were now available in the community. But frontline staff in both the secondary and community sectors claimed that the decision was misguided. Even one of my most circumspect respondents made the following observation:

> 'Ask anybody on the ground what the impact would be of shutting 38 medical beds and they would have told you it was asking for trouble.' I asked who made that decision and my respondent said that it was the Chief Executive 'because it was assumed that there would be facilities in the community to care for these patients but of course the facilities are not there'.

Clinicians repeatedly portrayed senior managers as lacking understanding of the situation confronting those at the frontline.

> She said that her colleague had asked in an open meeting whether there was a bed crisis and had been told emphatically by the Board Member that there was no bed crisis and the problem was an inability of the wards to discharge patients in a timely manner. Coordinator said, 'So there you go!' Coordinator said that the tone of the response was like that of a politician. She said this was frustrating as it was so far removed from reality. Another more senior nurse joined us at this point and while she stopped short of explicitly criticising the Board Member, she was evidently as unconvinced by the claim that there was no bed crisis. She said that this was based on findings 'according to some great computer'.

A senior nurse in the Emergency Unit told me that she had asked for additional resources to support the deployment of a nurse to care for patients in the corridor. Until a bed was found these were either the responsibility of the triage nurse, or paramedics were required to stay in the department. Her request was denied, however, because 'officially they did not have patients in the corridor'. It was also the case that senior level managers did not appreciate some of the difficulties faced by staff on the ground when confronted with the need to make a decision about the creation of extra capacity. As I have argued, such decisions were hugely consequential for the organisation as they entailed employing extra staff and possibly cancelling scheduled operations and they had to be taken in a dynamic and rapidly changing environment, where the available information was uncertain. If they did not act early enough to put in place a contingency plan then pressures increased in the Emergency Unit. If they acted prematurely, they could incur expenditure for the organisation which, with the benefit of hindsight turns out to be unnecessary. They did not have a crystal ball and it seemed to me that they were in a no-win situation. In the first extract, the site manager talks about having received criticism for not acting quickly enough to create additional capacity. In the second, she has anticipated excess demand and put in place the necessary arrangements to increase capacity but despite considerable and lengthy negotiations cannot find hospital employees to staff the unit and so has to use agency staff, a decision which has to be authorised by a higher level manager.

> Site Manager recounted a story about an incident a few weeks ago where she had come under heavy criticism. 'The Executive said that I didn't act quickly enough to open Paediatric Short Stay Surgical Unit. [...] I'd worked hard all day; I'd had nothing to eat and drink and three times before they had come in I'd been round with the Medical Director but they said I had not worked hard enough. I was very upset by that, I was.'

> Site Manager: 'What a waste of time. You want to sort things out early and I have been in there, you're in there and nurses are trying to find staff and now they say "no". It is so frustrating. You are criticised and you work hard and they can't find a nurse and you ask for Agency and they say "no". Irrespective of everything you have done to plan they say "no". [...] They want us to make decisions and then we can't act on them!'

Discussion

In the different organisational locales, in a multitude of ways, it was nurses who were largely responsible for the management of beds throughout the system. In undertaking this work they drew on and developed intricate and sophisticated local knowledge and social capital in order to negotiate the best fit between individual needs and extant capacity. In a context of limited resources, their practices were the primary mechanism through which service quality and organisational efficiency were mediated. The issue of bed capacity is a complex question. It is a perennial problem in a number of healthcare systems, particularly publicly-funded services, and has been much debated. In the UK, stories of the bed crisis recur regularly in the media and acute hospitals appear to be in a state of permanent calamity. Yet in the only sociological study of bed management to date, Green and Armstrong's (1993, 1995) respondents did not believe additional beds were the answer. Most appeared to consider that the advantages of extra resources was illusionary in so far as admission and discharge criteria seemed to change according to the availability of beds so that whatever the size of the overall bed stock, some form of rationing would be necessary. My findings lend support to this view. As I outlined in Chapter 1, nurses' organising work is shaped by their positioning in relation to two activity systems: the care of patients and care of the organisation. These intersect and can interfere with each other and their interrelations must be negotiated. So when patient 'pathways' are presented by policy makers as arrangements that are managed more-or-less well within organisations designed for this purpose, this is misleading. Indeed, viewed through the lens of nurses' organising practices, it is impossible to conceive of patient care and organisational structures as discrete entities. On the contrary, they are implicated in each other. Nurses sit at the intersection of these tensions and their organising work entails making the daily accommodations necessary in order to reconcile the needs of individual patients, with that of patient populations and the organisation as a whole. This is a general feature of nursing work, but these processes are clearly revealed at the critical moments in which staff endeavoured to secure a suitable match with a suitable bed. As we have seen, these processes involve adjustments to the bed, but also a reconfiguration of patients to bring about a suitable coupling. This echoes the observations of Green and Armstrong (1995: 749) that 'in short, it was less clinical decisions which produced the problem of bed shortages than bed shortages which influenced clinical decisions'. If bed availability increases then thresholds change. Thus, while as a society there are some fundamental questions to be asked about where we draw the line and what we are prepared to pay for, some form of rationing is inevitable and in the work they do in matching patients with beds on a day-to-day basis nurses fulfil a vital role in balancing the needs of the individual with the needs of the populations served. These accommodations were hugely consequential for the quality and safety of patient care, but also the efficiency of the organisation. In making strategic decisions about bed capacity, my findings point to the need for service managers to make better use of the local knowledge developed by frontline nurses in fulfilling this function and for nurses charged with this responsibility to be better supported by the organisation in making critical decisions in conditions of uncertainty.

The literature on bed management is limited, but it is widely recognised that there is a need for better access to information on bed occupancy and availability. A report by the NHS Executive found that in over 90 per cent of organisations, the information was obtained by telephoning the wards (Allder *et al.* 2010). The report recommends that IT systems should be provided to ensure timely and accurate information, but their implementation requires careful consideration. At Parklands as we have seen, information on planned discharges was centrally available, but widely regarded as inaccurate. This is partly because ward staff were often too stretched to update the database, and partly because it was used as a performance indicator and thus the content was managed to ensure a display of a well-organised ward rather than reflecting actual practices on the ground. These tensions need to be taken into account if the benefits of the investment of resources in such systems are to be realised. There is also a danger that access to information systems may reduce the contact bed managers have with ward nurses. While walking the wards to retain an overview of the bed state may look like an inefficient process, many decisions about patient placements were finely balanced, politically sensitive judgements. Bed managers' regular visits to the ward areas helped to smooth these processes. It was also the case, that daily visits from the patient access nurses were also a powerful mechanism through which ward staff were enrolled in bed management and helped mediate the tension between the interests of the organisation and those of individual units. Maintaining good relationships with unit staff was essential to the smooth functioning of the system and these regular conversations kept ward nurses aligned with the wider organisational agenda. While clinical services preferred to care for 'their' patients, at the same time most accepted the need for flexibility given the wider system pressures.

> We move down to Snowdrop Ward ((Surgical Ward)) where the ward manager greets the patient access nurse with the question: 'Hi [] – tell me what is happening to this service?'
>
> Patient Access Nurse: 'How do you mean?'
>
> Ward Manager: 'All these medical patients!'
>
> Patient Access Nurse: 'I've got 40 on trolleys downstairs waiting for beds!'
>
> Ward Manager: 'Really – have you? Alright then!'

Conclusion

In this chapter I have examined the work nurses do to assign patients to beds. I have argued that in a context of increased specialisation, it is by ensuring that people are allocated to the right bed with all the associated resources this brings that the actor networks associated with their trajectory of care most easily can be aligned. At Parklands, nurses at all levels of the organisation and in all parts of the service had some responsibility for match-making. This was challenging work, carried out in difficult circumstances in which nurses sought to balance the needs of individuals with the needs of the organisation. It is also important work, work that is hugely consequential for patient care and organisational effectiveness, but which was largely taken-for-granted. Despite the centrality of their contribution to the organisation and their detailed understanding of the situation at the frontline, however, nurses were largely excluded from strategic decision-making.

Notes

1 This is taken from Law, J. (1994) *Organizing Modernity*. Oxford, Blackwell.
2 Goodwin (1994) deploys this term to refer to 'the socially organized ways of seeing and understanding events that are answerable to the distinctive interests of a particular social group' (606).
3 CIWA refers to 'Clinical Institute Withdrawal Assessment' and is a common measure used in North America to assess and treat Alcohol withdrawal syndrome

and for alcohol detoxification. This clinical tool assesses 10 common withdrawal signs. A score of more than 15 points is associated with increased risk of alcohol withdrawal effects such as confusion. Interestingly, although the term CIWA was common currency to refer to particular types of patient, nobody could tell me what it referred to.

4 The use of emotive patient cases to gain a tactical advantage in competition for beds.

5 The Emergency Unit was divided into Resuscitation, Majors, Minors. Patients with serious problems who may require admission are seen in Majors. Minors dealt with patients who do not have life threatening complaints.

6 A facility which enables suitable patients to be admitted on the day of surgery, allowing them to remain at home the night before their operation and enables the hospital to use its beds in the most efficient way.

References

Allder, S., Silvester, K. and P. Walley (2010). 'Managing capacity and demand across the patient journey.' *Clinical Medicine* 10(1): 13–15.

Bagust, A., Place, M. and J.W. Ponsett (1999). 'Dynamics of bed use in accommodating emergency admissions: stochastic simulation model.' *BMJ* 319: 155–158.

Baillie, H., Wright, W., McLeod, A., Craig, N., Leyland, A., Drummond, N. and A. Boddy (1997). *Bed Occupancy and Bed Management*. Glasgow, Department of Public Health, University of Glasgow.

Comptroller and Auditor General (2000). *Inpatient Admissions and Bed Management in NHS Acute Hospitals*. London.

Dingwall, R. and T. Murray (1983). 'Categorization in accident departments: "good" patients, "bad" patients and "children".' *Sociology of Health & Illness* 5(2): 127–148.

Dr Foster Intelligence (2012). *Fit for the Future? Dr Foster Hospital Guide 2012*. London, Imperial College.

Goodwin, C. (1994). 'Professional Vision.' *American Anthropologist* 96(3): 606–633.

Green, J. and D. Armstrong (1993). 'Controlling the "bed state": negotiating hospital organization.' *Sociology of Health & Illness* 15(3): 337–352.

—— (1995). 'Achieving rational management: bed managers and the crisis in emergency admissions.' *Sociological Review* 43(4): 743–762.

Hillman, A. (2013). '"Why must I wait?" The performance of legitimacy in a hospital emergency department.' *Sociology of Health & Illness* 36(4): 485–499.

House of Commons (2010a). Independent Inquiry into Care Provided by Mid Staffordshire NHS Foundation Trust January 2005–March 2009 (Chaired by Robert Francis, QC). London, House of Common. 1.

—— (2010b). Independent Inquiry into Care Provided by Mid Staffordshire NHS Foundation Trust January 2005–March 2009 (Chaired by Robert Francis, QC). London, House of Common. 2.

Jeffery, R. (1979). '"Normal rubbish": deviant patients in causalty departments.' *Sociology of Health & Illness* 1(1): 90–107.

Keogh, B. (2013). *Review into the Quality of Care and Treatment Provided by 14 Hospital Trusts in England*. Overview Report, NHS.

Law, J. (1994) *Organizing Modernity*. Oxford, Blackwell.

Nugus, P., Bridges, J. and J. Braithwaite (2009). 'Selling patients.' *BMJ* 339: 5201.

Strauss, A., Fagerhaugh, S. and B. Suczet (1985) *The Social Organization of Medical Work*, Chicago, University of Chicago Press.

Vassy, C. (2001). 'Categorisation and micro-rationing: access to care in a French emergency department.' *Sociology of Health & Illness* **23**(5): 615–632.

Vygotsky, L. (1978). *Mind in Society: The Development of Higher Psychological Processes*. Cambridge, MA., Harvard University Press.

Walford, S. (2002). *Unexpected Medical Illness and the Hospital Response. Models of Emergency Care*. Warwick, University of Warwick.

5   Passing the baton, parsing the patient

Following a diagnosis of bowel cancer George Brown was admitted to hospital for surgery on 9 January 2012 and underwent an eight hour operation. Post-operatively he developed severe peritonitis and required admission to Intensive Care. Notwithstanding this complication, George eventually made a good recovery from his surgery and was able to be discharged home. On 28 February 2012 George was readmitted to hospital by his GP following an episode of breathlessness and light headedness. After spending some time in the Medical Assessment Unit, he was eventually admitted to the Coronary Care Unit with cardiac arrhythmias. After several days, in the light of George's conversations with members of his family, it became evident that the staff on the Coronary Care Unit had little information on George's previous surgery and as a consequence his nutritional and dietary requirements, all central to his post-operative recovery, had been overlooked. The family spoke to the nurse in the Coronary Care Unit who managed to locate and supply George with the supplementary energy drinks that he had been previously prescribed, and arranged for a nutritional assessment. This also precipitated the ward to organise meetings with the cardiac, surgical and oncology teams to discuss George's care. Had it not been for the family's intervention, George's needs in relation to his recent surgery would have been overlooked.[1]

As healthcare becomes ever-more specialised and bed pressures increase, patients typically traverse multiple services during an in-patient episode and such boundary crossings can have a significant influence on the care they receive. All handovers are error prone; and poorly managed they can lead to discontinuities and delays that create problems for patients, their families and organisations (Bryan et al. 2005). Unsurprisingly then, the effective navigation of service interfaces has been the focus of numerous improvement initiatives in recent years (Catchpole et al. 2007; Kripalani et al. 2007; Currie and Watterson 2008). Healthcare systems are an intricate matrix of interfaces of different kinds and the question of how best to manage transfers of care at specific boundary crossings might legitimately constitute a research study in its own right. In this chapter my purpose is not to undertake a detailed analysis of particular interfaces, but to describe in broad terms the everyday contribution of hospital nurses to transfers of care so that we might better understand this aspect of their work. At Parklands, all health providers contributed to interface management in some way, particularly as this related to inter-professional boundaries, but given their location in the sites of care and everyday contribution to the organisation of service delivery (Chapters 2 and 3), it was nurses who were largely charged with overall responsibility for this function. Managing transfers of care was a significant component of the workload of ward and unit nurses and, as we saw in the last chapter, at Parklands a number of specialist roles were dedicated to coordinating patient pathways. To some extent, navigating service interfaces called for the same organising work as that outlined in the previous chapters: match-making; accumulating, synthesising and translating information; initiating, aligning and integrating lines of work; and assembling the relevant constellations of material artefacts. I will not repeat these observations here. My concern in this chapter is to draw out a further major component of nurses' organising work which, while interleaved with these wider organising processes, is specific to transfers of care: parsing patients.

Rethinking transfers of care

> [E]ffective discharge from secondary care can be likened to the smooth flow in which the relay runners pass the baton over to the next runner. In a relay race you can't just throw the baton up in the air and hope the next person catches it. You must keep a firm hold of the baton until you are absolutely sure the next person has got it.
>
> (National Leadership and Innovation Agency
> for Healthcare 2008: 4)

Within the professional and policy literature, boundary crossing at departmental and organisational interfaces is generally conceptualised as a process in which responsibility for the care of a patient is transferred from one service to another, the success of which is believed to hinge on role clarity and accurate information exchange. Such assumptions are implicit in the title of the manual – 'Passing the Baton' (National Leadership and Innovation Agency for Healthcare 2008) – from which the above quote is taken. A practical guide for providers, the metaphor of the baton handover is intended to portray 'a seamless transfer of care' and to underline staff responsibilities in negotiating service interfaces, in this case hospital discharge. In order to understand the work nurses do in navigating departmental and organisational interfaces, we need first to rethink this accepted wisdom. I will show that navigating boundary crossings involves more than a clear division of labour and robust systems of knowledge management, it also requires the 'parsing' of patient identities. 'Parsing' is used here in the sense in which it is deployed in computing to refer to the process through which the course code of a computer program is analysed before it is turned into machine code. In healthcare, an analogous process takes place in navigating service interfaces in which, in order to secure a boundary crossing, patients must be translated from the work object of one service to the work object of another, and this requires that their identities are figured and reconfigured. It may be uncomfortable to think of people in this way – as work objects – and I am not suggesting that this is how providers orient to patients, but it does better describe the action that is necessary to accomplish service integration at critical interfaces. At Parklands it was nurses who were largely responsible for this work.

As I have argued in earlier chapters, people do not arrive in healthcare systems as ready-made work objects. Nurses have an important role at the gateways to the service in drawing together a range of information, signs and symptoms to assemble an organisational identity through which the person with an illness or injury is transformed into a patient and the relevant activity system set in train. But these are short-lived settlements. As the network of associated actors is mobilised, and individual and organisational interests seep into each other, trajectories evolve along distributed and largely independent parallel paths. The multiple versions of the patient that emerge from these processes are crystallised only briefly by momentary stabilisations arising from nurses' ongoing interactions with care providers and formal coordination events such as multidisciplinary team meetings. For much of the time, then, trajectories are an amorphous network of heterogeneous elements. When a decision is taken to transfer a patient from one department to another, however, greater solidity is required and this requires parsing work.

For the transferring department, a transfer of care is an occasion of closure in which the trajectory and its history must be crystallised, that is, formally brought together, and transformed. This is always a retrospective construction: the 'actors look back and review the entire course they have traversed' (Strauss 1985: 4) and the sense and meaning of a trajectory is accomplished once elapsed actions are available for review (also, see Berg 1992). But this transformation has another dimension. Beyond the work of reaching closure from the perspective of existing providers, transfers of care also require patients to be reassembled into the work object of the new service and identities must be (re)configured accordingly. Thus, transfers of care involve a double translation process and have a retrospective–prospective orientation. Boundary crossing requires staff to look back to figure patient identities in terms of the course that has been travelled and forward to translate this into a form that will facilitate their onward journey. Although they played a relatively minor role in their day-to-day management of trajectories, documents were significant actors for the purposes of interface management. They mediated the relationships between the different segments of the healthcare system and were a primary source of the paperwork about which nurses habitually complained.

Transfers of care are highly variable, and the source of this variability is both clinical and organisational. Patients have different levels of acuity and complexity of need. Thus the issues at stake when an acutely ill child attached to life-supporting technologies is transferred from operating theatres to the Intensive Care Unit are quite different from those associated with the transfer of care of a frail older person from an in-patient rehabilitation ward to a nursing home. Moreover, as Strauss (1985) recognised, progressing patient trajectories across service interfaces is also shaped by the relationship between collaborating sub-units and the extent to which they understand each other's work processes.

> Whether the work goes smoothly or conflictually is [...] first and foremost because the divergent lines of work characteristic of those different social worlds mix harmoniously or only with great tension and discord. The greater the discrepancy in social world perspective and activity, the more obviously will there be a need for explicit negotiation among workers to get the joint or collective tasks accomplished with any efficiency. If the workers have labored together previously and are now accustomed to working together, then they will have done the negotiative work previously; so, only new contingencies will bring about any awareness among them that negotiative work is again necessary.
>
> (Strauss 1985: 11)

These considerations all have a bearing on the challenges of boundary crossing, the arrangements that must be in place to support them and the work of nurses.

Crystallising trajectories and reconfiguring patients

Transfers of care across different service boundaries entailed work of different kinds and placed different demands on nurses on either side of the interface. It is impossible to do justice to this rich variety in a single chapter. I have insufficient data for this purpose and the study was not designed to undertake this kind of analysis.[2] In order to make visible this element of the nursing function, give a flavour of its variety and highlight some of the challenges involved, I have selected key illustrative examples of healthcare interfaces that were consequential for patient flows through the organisation. As with the rest of this book, in order to describe the work involved in parsing patients in each case it will also be necessary to consider the system features that give rise to it.

The first example we will look at is the interface between the Short Stay Surgical Unit and the operating theatres. Short Stay Surgical Units are a commonplace feature of the contemporary healthcare landscape and, when it was not being used as overflow for the rest of the hospital, the unit at Parklands was organised to run like a finely-tuned machine. Designed to care for a high volume of today's routine cases, it was founded on predictable recovery trajectories and rationalised processes. Here, as with many of the other elective surgical units, any investigations and assessments that were a prerequisite for theatre had been undertaken by specialist nurses prior to admission and quite possibly on the same day as the out-patients clinic appointment at which it had been decided that an operation was necessary. Thus when individuals arrived at the unit on the morning or afternoon of their procedure, much of the work of configuring their identities to transform them into the work object of the surgical team had already taken place. Managing the transfer of their care from the unit to the operating theatres entailed checking and finalising this process, referred to by the coordinator as 'sort(ing) out their notes'.

> I asked Coordinator what the nurses managing a list would do. She said that they would collect the patient from Reception and bring them to their bed, instruct them about getting into a gown and then 'sort out their notes'. The latter includes ensuring they have a signed consent form, forms for TTHs ((tablets to take home)), a sick note if they require one ((signed by the surgeon in theatres)), checklist for theatre, details of next of kin and their telephone number, GP details, plus information on health, allergies etc. They would then 'check their obs' ((make recordings of vital signs)). When they are happy that everything is in order they enter their details into Theatre Man ((an IT system)) which notifies theatres that the patient is ready.

In this context 'sorting out their notes' involved several interleaved tasks. It entailed action to assemble the artefacts designed to prompt and facilitate the work of theatre staff and ensure trajectory articulation – such as the forms on which the surgeon will prescribe tablets for the patient to take home and a sick note to be signed if the patient requires it. But it also involves work to ensure the completion of all relevant documentation through which patient identities are configured for the work purposes of operating theatres. This is a highly selective representation of the patient and reflects operating theatre work. So while it is important to know about the existence of allergies, when the patient last ate, their weight, and whether they have dental caps or crowns, no information is included about their social circumstances, their mobility, hobbies, community support networks, dietary preferences or any of the other details which make up individuals and might be relevant in addressing other facets of their care needs. These aspects of patients' identities are not relevant for the work of theatre staff. Moreover, much of this information was already available as a result of the great deal of preparatory work undertaken in out-patients clinic by the anaesthetic pre-assessment nurses in which an individual's fitness for surgery had been established. Thus a considerable amount of effort has already been undertaken at this interface to progressively shape individuals to be amenable to the requirements of the surgical team. Parsing patients on the day of their procedure required Short Stay Surgical Unit nurses to make sure the documentation to accompany them to theatre was in order. In fulfilling this function they were guided by a checklist which precisely specified the information required.

Once the paperwork was assembled, the ward nurse notified theatres electronically and staff then collected the patient with little or no interaction with the unit nurses. Here, then, boundary crossing was achieved through the checklist which functioned as a translation device to mediate the interface between departments and enabled the effective processing of a high volume of cases each day and ensured nothing was missed and that the operation could proceed safely. We might think of this as a technically mediated transfer of care, made possible by the work done before admission in which an individual's fitness for surgery has been established and the prior work that has gone into the carefully designed documentation which specified the information required on the day of surgery to support patient flows. It is an example of what is referred to in ANT as black-boxing, in which a technology becomes taken-for-granted and the complex socio-material relationships that constitute it are rendered invisible. Many healthcare interfaces cannot be managed in this way, however, and successful boundary crossing depends on more complex arrangements. The transfer of care between Theatre Recovery and the surgical wards is a case in point.

Operating theatres are an expensive organisational resource and maximising their use is an important priority for the acute sector. Following surgery all patients require post-anaesthetic care before they can be returned to the wards. If beds are unavailable in Recovery then patients have to remain in theatres creating delays in the schedule and possibly cancelled operations after patients have been admitted. If patients leave the unit before they are physiologically stable then their safety is put in jeopardy and so too is that of others if ward nurses are distracted by the requirement to manage an unstable or at risk patient. Like the previous example, this interface was mediated by a complex constellation of artefacts central to which was a handover checklist that functioned as a translation device and required the recovery nurse to demonstrate that the patient was fit for transfer. The retrospective–prospective translation involved in this process is evident in the following extract. Recovery nurses work on a one-to-one basis with patients and during her time in the unit the patient's vital signs have been continuously monitored using an electronic device. Having attended closely to her patient, the recovery nurse is satisfied that she is physiologically stable and can leave the unit. When I join her at the bedside she is completing the paperwork which will accompany the woman back to the ward.

> Staff Nurse is recovering a patient in the space directly opposite the Nurses' Station. She is completing paperwork and as I approach she says that she is 'getting up to date with the observation charts' before

she takes the patient back to the ward. She is filling in an 'arterial observations' chart, completing the information on a host of clinical indicators for a series of 15 minutely observations which she has not yet recorded hard copy. After she has completed this documentation she moves on to the observations ((BP, Temp, pulse)) chart. Here again she goes through the same process of completing the form but this time using information from the monitor to update the information. She explained that the monitor recorded blood pressure every five minutes but that they only recorded it on the observations chart every fifteen minutes. The monitor can provide a record of all the patient's vital signs whilst they have been in Recovery ((this information is cleared when they are discharged back to the wards)). When she has done this she ticks all the boxes in the 'recovery discharge criteria' checklist, which includes inter alia: maintenance of airway, oxygen saturation, respiratory rate, cardiovascular observations, temperature, surgical drains, wound site, pain, urine output, neurological status, nausea and vomiting.

In this example, the nurse brings about a retrospective crystallisation and prospective translation of the patient's identity narrowly defined in terms of the physiological parameters of recovery and which is formally mediated by a handover checklist and the associated observational charts. This paperwork brings together the numerous physiological observations through which the nurse has reached a decision about the patient's suitability for transfer, enables her to account for her own action by documenting the parameters of the patient's recovery and to demonstrate through the satisfactory completion of the discharge criteria the patient's readiness to leave the unit. Through this process the individual is transformed from a patient recovering from anaesthesia to a patient suitable for transfer. Then, having assembled this information and completed the handover checklist, the nurse accompanies the patient back to the ward.

> Recovery Nurse is telling the patient that she is back on the ward now. Staff Nurse 1 checks her temperature and reads out the observations from the monitor to Staff Nurse 2 who records them on the observation chart. Recovery Nurse is telling Staff Nurse 1 about the Patient Controlled Analgesia ((PCA)) and the fact that it is a high dose. She informs the nurse that the Pain Team will come and see the patient.
>
> Recovery Nurse: 'She's been pressing away. She knows she needs to wait for the light to come on but it's difficult for her to see it. Her blood ((transfusion)) is due to run out about ten to five.'
>
> Staff Nurse 1 looks at the clock; it is 16:30.
>
> Recovery Nurse: 'She has another ((unit of blood)) to go through two to three hourly. The anaesthetist signed this ((for the blood)) by mistake.

((Both nurses are looking at the chart)). I can vouch for her signature; it is the same as it is written down there. I've written error.'

Recovery Nurse asks Staff Nurse 1 if she wants her 'to take her through her wound sites'. Staff Nurse 1 says she does and they draw the curtains around the patient's bed. I retreat to the ward corridor.

After the patient has been settled in her bed Recovery Nurse asks Staff Nurse 1 if she would like to handover. They walk down to the Nurses' Station. Recovery Nurse asks Staff Nurse 1 if she knows the patient. She does not. Recovery Nurse explains that the patient has been rather difficult whilst in Recovery and that she had initially been concerned that it was the effects of the anaesthetic. However, she then recalled having cared for the patient previously and on this occasion she had been equally abrasive. She explains that her irritability had been triggered by the Recovery Nurse mispronouncing the patient's unusual name. She observes that the patient is a nurse and wants to do things herself. Having had this discussion, Recovery Nurse hands over more formally.

Recovery Nurse: 'She's had a right fem pop by-pass and has been on regular vascular obs and analgesia as required.'

She talks about medications given in theatre and explains that she has a PCA running.

Recovery Nurse: 'I gave her a couple of bolus doses of morphine and she would fall asleep and then wake up in pain again so I've put her on the PCA. She's had Hartmann's in theatre to try and keep her blood pressure up and its now trickling through with the PCA. She's had nothing for sickness and has been settled. I've taken her arterial line out. She has a grey venflon with blood going through and a pink venflon with the PCA.'

Staff Nurse 1: 'So fluids are going through the PCA?'

Recovery Nurse: 'Yeah a trickle through at eight hourly. Her last BM was 4.2 and I've left her on 3 litres of oxygen. Her temperature is quite low – 35.4 – but it's been consistent. She's self-medicating. She apparently refused a sliding scale insulin saying she wanted to manage her own medications and had [...] units this morning which is stupid.'

Staff Nurse 1: 'She should know better.'

The nurses then discuss the fact that the patient had taken her tablets which lower blood pressure and her blood pressure has also been low during surgery. The two nurses discuss the foolhardiness of these decisions and express surprise given the patient's clinical background. Recovery Nurse asks Staff Nurse 1 if she would like to sign the care plan to show she has accepted her back. This she does.

The handover in this example falls into distinct sections. The centrepiece is a formal presentation of facts about the patient's operation, subsequent care in Recovery and ongoing requirements, and has a ceremonial format. It covers most of the issues itemised in the handover checklist and which are documented in the medical record, but includes wider contextual and interpretative information. For example, the nurse explains the decision-making process which led to the patient being prescribed patient controlled analgesia ('I gave her a couple of bolus doses of morphine and she would fall asleep and then wake up in pain') and also accounts for the fact that she has Hartmann's solution intravenously ('She's had Hartmann's in theatre to try and keep her blood pressure up and its now trickling through with the PCA'). This formal handover is enfolded in a wider narrative account of the patient's behaviours and the challenges the recovery nurse has encountered caring for her and an evaluative discussion about the patient's refusal to follow medical advice in relation to her insulin management. It is a nice illustration of the work nurses do in tailoring trajectory narratives according to the needs of the audience and in this case, includes information relevant to the receiving nurses' work purposes – the patient is known to be an irascible character – and which is unlikely to be readily available in the patient record. A further interesting feature of this extract is that the recovery nurse also offers contextual information necessary for interpretation of the patient's prescription charts whereby she explains to the ward nurse that a unit of blood has been signed for in error.

Despite the centrality of artefacts in mediating the transfer process, in this example a human mediator is also necessary to bring about the required translations to ensure a safe handover. Illustrating the work nurses do in taking the perspective of others (see Chapter 2), the theatre recovery nurse provides important contextual information that is an essential background for the purposes of interpreting the formal written record which is relevant to the work purposes of the ward nurse and will eventually be incorporated into this patient's trajectory narrative. Many artefacts in healthcare can be understood as 'designated boundary objects' (Levina and Vaast 2005), that is objects that have been identified or indeed developed as valuable for boundary spanning. However, these only become 'boundary objects-in-use' if the artefacts are both meaningfully incorporated into the local practices of different groups while acquiring a common identity in the context of joint practices (Levina and Vaast 2005). Here the recovery nurse fulfils a boundary spanning role which activates the boundary spanning capacity of the documentation by providing the necessary contextual information the ward nurse requires to interpret the forms.

In the two examples considered thus far, we have focused on the patient parsing work of nurses in the originating unit. But nurses in the receiving service also had a role in bringing patients into the local work organisation. Transfers of care varied according to the balance of retrospective–prospective translational work required and its distribution between the nurses in the respective units or departments. Thus in the example of the transfer of care from the Short Stay Surgical Unit to operating theatres the demands on the receiving department were minimal, and the onus was on unit staff to pre-configure patients for theatre. But in other kinds of boundary crossing, typically those between wards within the hospital, the obligation was on the receiving department to bring the patient into their local work organisation. In principle, the referring department was responsible for trajectory crystallisation prior to transfer but there was no formal documentation through which this was mediated and handover in such cases was typically oral – either face-to-face or over the telephone – and, to a considerable extent, depended on the current trajectory narrative in circulation (see Chapter 2), rather than formal processes of documentation, other than the requirement to indicate transfer had taken place. Thereafter, ward nurses would take responsibility for assembling the constellation of artefacts through which patients were brought into the work organisation of the receiving departments. This next example arises from my observations on a surgical ward and relates to a transfer of care from the Surgical Assessment Unit.

> Staff Nurse 1 has had a new admission from the Surgical Assessment Unit. She is looking through his notes to see if all the information she needs is there. She adds the existing pile of notes to the ward admission booklet and transfers face-sheet data and a few details onto this form.
>
> Later on in the shift I observe her completing the standard post-operative care plan for this patient. Presumably no post-operative care plan has come with him from Surgical Assessment Unit. She is adding in the date, signing some of the care plan sections and crossing out others. She has added to his notes a falls risk form, a Pat-e-Bac assessment ((manual handling risk assessment)), a stool chart and a daily observations chart. She spots a VIPs ((Venous Infusion Phlebitis form, a quality intervention designed to ensure intravenous sites are reviewed regularly to reduce infections caused by peripheral venous cannulae)) form on the desk and says 'I'll have one of those'.
>
> Staff Nurse 2: 'Are you pinching the one I left out?'
>
> Staff Nurse 1: 'I saw it there and thought "I'll have one of those", I forgot to put one in.'
>
> Staff Nurse 2: 'Just as well I had a spare one!'

At ward level, this kind of scenario was repeated on a frequent basis as nurses assembled the materials through which patients were figured and reconfigured as the work object for different departments. As we saw in Chapter 3, this is one of the indirect mechanisms through which nurses endeavour to assign and articulate the diverse lines of activity that constitute trajectories of care. How far the artefacts successfully achieved this function is, I have argued, questionable. But these are the materials through which patients are made up (Hacking 2004, 2007) and are required to be in place in order that care can be accounted for and quality evidenced; and it was time-consuming work. Several wards had preassembled bundles of artefacts which were used to admit new patients and included all the requisite checklists and risk assessment forms. This obviated the need for *de novo* decisions about the materials required in each case, but there was still effort involved in tailoring these to the requirements of individuals.

Ward nurses also undertook considerable work in parsing patients for the purposes of discharge planning which, unlike internal transfers of care, entailed more formalised processes. As we have seen, for all its gloss of rationality and team talk, healthcare work is but loosely coupled and, for much of the time, trajectories are largely formless phenomena. It is through their knowledge creation and trajectory articulation work that nurses bring about the necessary translations through which network actors are aligned in order for patient care to be progressed. Notwithstanding the inherent centrifugal tendencies in these arrangements, I have argued for their necessity in affording flexibility in organising healthcare work in a context of multiple and uncertain demands and in overcoming the limitations of the medical record in supporting knowledge and information flows for the purposes of everyday healthcare delivery. However, this presents significant challenges in reaching closure when care must be navigated across departmental and organisational interfaces. In the example of transfers from theatre recovery to the surgical wards, the trajectory in question is relatively short and the relevant details confined to those pertaining to the immediate peri- and post-operative periods, much of which is pre-specified in the handover checklist. Whereas, when a patient is discharged from the ward the trajectory details are far more wide-ranging and their relevance to the patient's onward journey less clearly-defined.

In the next section I look at a fairly simple example: the transfer of care from hospital to community nursing services. At Parklands this was mediated by a transfer letter, a comparatively unstructured document which allowed free-text entries under topic headings, reflecting the broad range of patients and purposes to which the documents were intended to apply. Compared to the work entailed in filling out the checklists that mediated the interfaces between wards, recovery and operating theatres, completion of the community nursing referral documentation obliged nurses to exercise rather more judgement about what information to include or not. They were required to assume the perspective of the community nursing service and anticipate their information needs in order that they could successfully take over the patient's care. My observations with the community nursing service revealed that secondary sector staff sometimes struggled to do this. Unlike internal transfers of care within the hospital, which could be facilitated by face-to-face handover, this was not the case with the community service and the discharge letter was intended to fulfil this purpose on its own. It did not always succeed, however. When I shadowed the community nurses, I saw several examples in which it was necessary for them to contact ward-based staff to clarify the details in a given case and my conversations with them indicated that this was not an uncommon occurrence, particularly in relation to specialist procedures and technologies which, while the routine business of secondary care specialists, were unfamiliar to the community services.

Patient transfers to the community nursing services centred on delimited issues, such as wound care, and were nurse-to-nurse handovers. The challenges of boundary crossing are further magnified when the responsibilities in question are more diffuse, where professional boundaries must be crossed and the departments on either side of the boundary are unknown to each other. Health and social care in the community is provided by a mixed economy of services; a patchwork quilt of private carers, local authority teams and nursing and residential homes. As we have seen, all have different referral criteria, the details of which are often opaque. Moreover, as social science has shown us, individuals' requirements for care are context dependent. The arrangements necessary to support someone in their own home are quite different from those that suffice in the acute care setting. As well has having an uncertain understanding of the requirements of the receiving service and the needs of patients in a new context, very often transfers of care have to be undertaken when there are few opportunities for face-to-face interaction. Thus, while the post-anaesthetic recovery nurse takes the patient back to the ward and hands over to the nurse who will be responsible for their continuing care, when a patient is transferred to a nursing or residential home they are accompanied by the ambulance service who have had no ongoing trajectory involvement. In such circumstances boundary crossing is heavily dependent on artefacts and, if documents are to travel between distant social worlds, then considerable elaboration is necessary and this can be a source of exasperation to the original community (Brown and Duguid 1996). In the study site, transfers of care from the hospital to the community, where input from social care agencies was required, were mediated by the unified assessment form. This was a lengthy document which was almost universally despised by hospital staff. Different providers had responsibility for completing different sections on the form but nurses were charged with the lion's share of this work.

> Coordinator: 'Of all the things we do I hate Unified Assessments. I sound like an old sceptic but I am not sure whether nursing was consulted and, if we are expected to fill things in, then we should have been.'

The underlying idea of the unified assessment form was to make available a summary of the patient's needs in a standardised format in order to support transfers of care from the secondary to the community care setting. As I have argued, all transfers of care require patient identities to be parsed so that they are compatible with the work of the receiving service and, as we saw in the previous chapter, in a context of securing a match under conditions of resource constraint, patient identities were also carefully crafted so that they met the referral criteria of the service. Because the documentation was based on a de-contextualised notion of patient 'need', it did little to orient ward staff to the translations required to ensure that the patient identities were presented in a form suitable for the work purposes of the community sector.

Given the broad population of patients to whom the form applied, the wide range of services to which patients were transferred, and the politicised context in which many hospital discharges were accomplished, ward staff struggled to complete the documentation satisfactorily. They were insufficiently familiar with the community care setting to appreciate the patient information required to support their work processes nor did they always understand the artistry involved in fabricating patient identities in order to secure a match (see Chapter 4). Thus in order for the unified assessment form to function successfully in mediating the relationship between health and social care, the discharge liaison nurses had an important role in assisting ward staff in making the necessary translations to expedite knowledge flows at this interface.

> Senior Nurse said that sometimes the ward nurses seemed to assume that other people had access to their background knowledge and so would know what was meant by written information. However, often this needs translating further so that other professionals fully understand the issues.

> Discharge Liaison Nurse locates a set of notes and leafs through a unified assessment form which has been completed. [...] She complains that the information provided is insufficient and more details are required. In one section it simply states that a patient is incontinent of urine and faeces. Discharge Liaison Nurse says that this needs to include information on how this is managed. [...] She said that one of the challenges for her was that there was a lack of understanding at ward level of the information that was required. Having looked through the unified assessment form Discharge Liaison Nurse makes an entry into the patient's notes requesting that more information is included and asks the ward to bleep her if they wish so that she can go through this with them.

Whereas the recovery nurse operated in a boundary spanning role to provide the necessary contextual information through which the handover document could be understood by ward staff, in this case, in which the opportunities for face-to-face interaction were limited, the discharge liaison nurse fulfilled an analogous function in order to ensure that the documentation was completed satisfactorily in order that it could successfully operate as a translation device in mediating the hospital-community interface.

In the examples so far considered, I have shown that transfers of care placed different demands on nurses in different parts of the system but common to all was agreement that the transfers were considered appropriate by both parties, and the division of labour between the participating departments was well-understood. As we saw in the previous chapter, however, in many cases transfers of care at the secondary–community interface are confounded by resource constraints and questions of financial responsibility and in such circumstances documents can also be used to police and control. In this context, the retrospective–prospective stabilisation of patient identities also becomes a politicised case-making process and the site of struggles about who is to pay. In such circumstances documents become boundary negotiating artefacts (Lee 2007).

Beyond the kinds of work involved in making a case outlined in the previous chapter, transfers of care involving patients who were considered to be eligible for continuing healthcare funding, also entailed an elaborate additional assessment process using a 'Decision Support Tool', which required the participation of the patient and/or their family. If considered to meet the criteria, the costs of their ongoing care would be funded by the health service; if not, they would be deemed in need of social care, which was means-tested. Although the final decision could not be contested, the procedure could. Thus nurses were at pains to ensure and document due process. This work fell to the discharge liaison nurses and was decidedly onerous.

> Discharge Liaison Nurse: 'The ward nurses perceive this job is cushy as "I sit in the office all day", but then I give them the pack I have prepared for the discharges and they are amazed by the size of it.'

The process of fabricating patient identities for the purposes of making an application for continuing healthcare entailed extensive documentation of the full extent of patient care needs, and was predicated on a deficit model which for patients and their families could be distressing.

> Discharge Liaison Nurse then talked about how completing the Decision Support Tool with patients can be quite distressing for them as it is focused on what they cannot do. She said that she tries to meet with them beforehand to forewarn them of this. She recounted an incident with one patient who got half way through the meeting and was getting distressed and said: 'I don't want to finish this – I've had enough.' Discharge Liaison Nurse: 'It's very hard as they are still coming to terms with what has happened to them.' She told me another story about a son who had wanted access to his mother's Decision Support Tool and Discharge Liaison Nurse had agreed to allow him to see it with the proviso that his mother agreed. She had also forewarned him about its focus and content and he came back to her and said: 'I am glad you forewarned me because I didn't recognise my mother in this.' I asked

whether he meant that he didn't agree with the assessment. Discharge Liaison Nurse: 'No, he knew she had problems, but seeing it written down like this had really brought it home.'

Not only does this example make visible a tremendously burdensome aspect of nurses' work in accomplishing transfers of care, it also reinforces the challenge laid down at the beginning of this chapter in relation to conventional assumptions about the handover process, and reveals very powerfully the work involved in the selective representation of patient identities and how their fabrication for the purposes of negotiating eligibility for funding sit uneasily with family members' perceptions of their loved ones.

Challenges

The work involved in parsing patients is highly variable across service interfaces as are the associated challenges, which makes summative statements difficult. Nevertheless, several common issues emerge from the examples considered here. First, as I have argued in Chapter 2, the growing requirement for transparency and accountability in healthcare has created increasingly complex systems of documentation, such that information about patients' care and treatment has become ever-more detailed but increasingly fragmented and hence more difficult to locate and summarise. For the practical purposes of service delivery, healthcare providers depended largely on the working knowledge created through the trajectory narratives circulated by nurses. The inadequacies of the medical record for supporting information flows are equally relevant for understanding the work involved in effecting the trajectory crystallisations necessary to support transfers of care, but in many instances, because face-to-face interaction is not possible, trajectory narratives cannot be relied upon. In the next example, the staff nurse is assembling the necessary information in order to complete the community nurse transfer letter.

> Staff Nurse is looking through the unified assessment form for the purposes of finding information to include in the community nurse transfer letter. Most of the booklet is blank – only the face sheet data is included. She flicks through the pages in a cursory manner. She is about to transfer the phone number when she notices that it has too many digits in it. She goes to the computer to cross-check and discovers that this is completely different, so she goes to speak to the patient. She returns, picks up the patient's notes and scrutinises the casualty card. She does not make any further entries into the transfer letter but leafs through the continuation sheets. She picks up her handover sheet from the desk and scrutinises this. She then enters information on the transfer letter in relation to past medical history which she has evidently been able to obtain from the handover sheet. She then moves on to scrutinise

the discharge notification form and extracts further information which she includes in the transfer letter.

Whilst she is doing this she answers the phone twice. On one occasion the call is from a social worker and she passes it to her colleague who is sitting next to her also writing her notes. The second call is an enquiry after a patient being cared for by someone else. He is not at the Nurses' Station and Staff Nurse has to leave the area to locate him. A few minutes later a medical consultant arrives on the ward and asks to see a patient. Staff Nurse directs him to the 9-bedded area. He asks for the patient's notes and she points to the notes trolley.

Catching sight of the deputy ward manager who is passing through the Nurses' Station, Staff nurse asks: 'Do you remember with Pat's wound, did it dehis[3] or did it just open?'

DWM(L): 'It didn't dehis, it just gradually opened over a few days and we got more and more packing in.'

This typical example reveals the work and some of the challenges involved in stabilising trajectories for the purposes of effecting transfers of care. We can see that the nurse does not rely exclusively on the main body of the medical record (continuation sheets), but endeavours to locate the information required from other summative documents – the unified assessment form (which has not been completed), the casualty card (completed in the Emergency Unit on admission), the notification of discharge form (completed by the junior doctors who use it to prescribe the medications for discharge) – as well as drawing on her personal trajectory narrative plot summary (handover sheet), the patient themselves and a colleague – to piece together the information required. This was time-consuming work.

It is also the case that in fulfilling this function the nurse is interrupted three times. This was not an unusual scenario as nurses typically completed transfer documentation either at the Nurses' Station where they were able to access the medical record or at the bedside, which rendered them liable to interruptions. For example, when I shadowed the surgical unit coordinator managing a theatre list, she had to stop her work of 'sorting out the notes' on several occasions in order that others could attend to the patient.

Coordinator returns to patient 1 ((a young woman with fertility problems)) and starts working through the details on the pre-assessment booklet to check that everything is completed. [...] As she is attending to the patient, the anaesthetist arrives and wants to do the pre-anaesthetic assessment. Coordinator leaves the anaesthetist to talk to the patient but remains behind the curtains attending to her paperwork. A little later the surgeon arrives. Coordinator decides to leave the doctors to get on with their tasks. Leaving the patient, Coordinator says to me: 'See what I mean about not being able to get on. And she's first on the list.'

At the time of the study, when nurses at Parklands dispensed medications they wore red tabards inscribed with a 'do not disturb' instruction – an intervention designed to reduce interruptions and thus medication errors (Scott *et al.* 2010). Medication rounds are very visible work with self-evident implications for patient safety and while there is little evidence in support of the effectiveness of tabards in reducing interruptions and medication errors (Raban and Westbrook 2013), the important point for current purposes is that the risks associated with interruptions are recognised. Completing paperwork for the purpose of transfers of care is a less obviously risky task but the consequences of getting this wrong are no less significant. Discharge liaison nurses completed this work in the relative calm of their admittedly over-crowded offices, but ward nurses were expected to do the same in the turbulence of the clinical environment. This raises the issue as to whether designated spaces that are free from interruptions should be made available in the sites of care where nurses can undertake patient parsing work.

As we have seen, documents were central actors in negotiating transfers of care and in some of the examples considered here they functioned very effectively to parse patients at service interfaces. We saw how the formal handover checklists mediated the relationship between operating department and the wards so that at the point of transfer patient identities were strongly prefigured for the work purposes of the receiving department. Transfers between wards and units were rather looser arrangements, however, with little requirement for pre-configuration on the part of the transferring department. Furthermore, handover in most cases was accomplished through social interaction, either face-to-face or by telephone. Given the pressures on beds within the organisation, nurses often received little notice of imminent transfers and with no formal mechanisms for parsing patients, individuals could be moved on before the work necessary to crystallise a given trajectory narrative had been undertaken. Flows of patients could thus outstrip flows of information or put slightly differently, patient bodies could arrive on a unit before a stabilisation of their identities has been reached. In the following example, a nurse from the surgical assessment unit has arrived on the ward to transfer a patient, but has a poor understanding of the details of her care. Here then, in a process which has parallels with the collaborative production of trajectory narratives described in Chapter 2, the nurses work together to make sense of and assemble a picture of the case.

> I observed the Surgical Assessment Unit nurse handover the patient, but her knowledge of the details of the case was extremely shaky. '[name] 52, came in with rigors and cellulitis on her back.' She stops and is flicking through the notes for more information but seems unable to locate it. 'She's on [name of drug] so she must have some gastric issues.' Both

nurses are now scrutinising the notes. 'She's on IV antibiotics and oral antibiotics. Her IV's been stopped...' She resumes looking at the notes. 'When I came on this morning she was off the ward and not back until 10am. She told me she had taken two Paracetamol. I've just done her obs and they are fine. She's apyrexial. Otherwise fine ((showing observation chart)).' Spotting something on the chart 'Ah [?] that's why she's on [name of drug]. You need to check if she's epileptic if she takes this regularly as it is not written up. Where her cellulitis is drying out it is beginning to crack and I have asked the doctor to write her up for some cream.'

Although nurses understood these service pressures; inadequate handovers were subject to much criticism as in such cases the onus fell on the receiving department to build up a retrospective picture of the patient before they could configure identities for their own purposes and set into circulation the narratives to support trajectory mobilisation. It also presented potential risks to the quality and safety of patient care if vital information was omitted.

As I have argued, departments are becoming increasingly specialised, but they also face pressures to improve and demonstrate the quality of their services. Documents are one of the mechanisms through which this was achieved and a striking finding of this study was the extent to which the different services within Parklands had their own singular artefacts for managing work processes. As I have argued, documents are an important means through which organisations can secure legitimacy and current approaches to quality improvement encourage these trends. As a consequence, however, each transfer of care required information to be entered into the new forms and formats of the receiving department. The following extract is taken from my observations in the Medical Assessment Unit in which a nurse educator is supporting a student nurse to complete the unit's documentation on a patient who has been transferred from the Emergency Unit.

> I resume observing the student nurse and unit educator. The Educator is looking at the completed paperwork and praises student nurse for her front sheet. 'This is one of the best I've seen. The only thing missing is the telephone number of the next of kin but I appreciate it can be difficult. But we're doing an audit on these to see what information is recorded.' The Educator then moves on to complete the other components of the Medical Assessment Unit booklet. She tells the student nurse that she finds it easier to transfer the information from the Emergency Unit records to the Medical Assessment Unit records. She transfers this information and puts a line across the Emergency Unit paperwork. This is one of many occasions in which I observed nurses transferring information from one record keeping format to another or assembling information in different ways for different purposes. I clarified with the Educator that I had correctly understood what she had done and [...] she confirmed my interpretation.

Assembling the appropriate constellation of documents that bring patients into the local work organisation was a major component of the nursing workload. It was also a source of some frustration.

> Staff Nurse observed that 'this pen pushing was ridiculous'. He said that the ward was very busy and that they were often run off their feet and the excessive paperwork added to this and took them away from the patients. He talked too about the different forms and booklets associated with the different departments in the hospital and the time involved in copying and transferring information from one format to another. [...] He said 'If it's all the same paperwork it's OK. Transferring patients from Green Ward is OK as they use the same documentation. But they have a pink form from Surgical Assessment Unit and a huge yellow one from the Medical Assessment Unit.'

> Coordinator: 'But you have to be hot on the paperwork as if it's not documented then it's not done. Then we've got all these new things like VIPS ((Venous Infusion Phlebitis form)) and the skin bundle ((a quality initiative in which a group of interventions are brought together to ensure pressure area care; it requires documented interventions, 2 hourly)).'

Not only was this a enormously time-consuming activity, it also carried very real risks to quality and safety as at each boundary crossing information could become lost in translation. As my earlier example showed, the nurse who was trying to complete the paperwork necessary for a transfer of care discovered two different phone numbers recorded for the patient, neither of which was correct. Furthermore, because of the sheer volume of documentation involved in parsing patients, the purpose and importance of the work becomes rather lost. In a number of the examples presented here, nurses referred to the process as one of 'sorting out the paperwork', signalling a drift towards a culture in which the paperwork becomes the end rather than the means. There was clear evidence of this in the case of transfers of care from the wards to the community, where staff regarded completion of the unified assessment form as burdensome bureaucracy rather than a mechanism for safeguarding follow-on care.

> Discharge Liaison Nurse said that the Unified Assessments took about four hours to complete if they were done properly and she could understand why the wards did not complete them well. 'It is a big form and ward staff see it as a task.'

It was also the case that, within the hospital, the medical record comprised of a substantial body of documentation, much of which was not completed.

> It was quiet and so I leafed through another set of notes. Here I noticed that there is a pink 'surgical admissions' booklet. Most of the sections

were not completed – such as the section for the medical clerking – where there was a note which read: see admission clerking on separate history sheet. The trouble with the integrated booklets is that they can only be used by one person at a time. Other sections left blank were: PMH ((past medical history)), current medications, social history.

Discussion

As we have seen, transfers of care vary in their complexity and make different demands on participants before knowledge can be shared. Ward nurses bear the brunt of the responsibility for this work, and as patient throughput increases so does the work involved. Factors that are consequential for this work include the complexity and predictability of patient trajectories, the range of trajectory types traversing an interface, the scope of care responsibility to be handed over, the proximity and familiarity of collaborating departments/professions, the amenability of the transfer process to rationalisation and technical mediation, the scope for boundary crossing to be supported by social interaction, the degree of interpretative work demanded of practitioners in fabricating identities for the work purposes of others, the ease with which pertinent information can be accessed and the politics of transfer. Thus transfers between proximal units within the organisation were easier to effect than transfers that entailed connecting more distant departments which interacted infrequently. The management of internal transfers of care which could be supported by human mediation were generally less demanding than those involving external agencies where the scope for face-to-face interaction was more limited. And transfers where relevant patient identities could be rationalised and pre-specified were more amenable to black-boxed technical mediation than those in which the required information was more difficult to determine and involved sensemaking and interpretative work on the part of health professionals. Finally, it is clear that when the challenges of interface management are confounded by struggles over who is to pay, finding a match and securing a boundary crossing can be immeasurably more difficult and resource consuming.

Carlile (2002, 2004) argues that organisational interfaces can be categorised according to the challenges they present for knowledge-sharing and identifies three main types: 'syntactic' boundaries where the focus is on knowledge as something to capture, store and then transfer and which resonates with the Short Stay Surgical Unit example considered here; 'semantic' boundaries where the focus is on culture and the requirements of social interaction in translating knowledge before it can be shared and which has parallels with our post-anaesthetic recovery unit to surgical ward interface; and 'pragmatic' boundaries where the interface is political and contested, such as those transfers of care complicated by funding issues. He argues that the value of such a framework is that it enables us to think about the relative complexity of different boundaries and the implications this has for the infrastructural arrangements required for managing knowledge across them. For current purposes, it also provides a framework through which the burden of patient parsing work in a given unit might be assessed in order to inform workforce planning. The weight of work in relation to the management of transfers of care that confronts nurses working on a medical unit required to handle a highly variable patient population and interact with a wide range of services, is considerably greater than that required of specialist units dealing with planned admissions.

There is a sense in which Carlile's analysis presupposes that the complexity of a knowledge boundary exists independently of the infra-structural arrangements that are in place to support its management. It is possible to argue, however, that transfers of care are not inherently simple or complex; rather they reflect the degree of rationalisation that has taken place, the ease with which this can be achieved and the costs and benefits of undertaking such work. Thus while there is a case for investing in the development of an infrastructure to technically mediate transfers of clearly delimited populations with relatively predictable trajectories of care, in locales where individual patients are highly variable and their trajectories emergent this becomes more difficult. In such cases, rather than searching for a technical fix, interface management may best be accomplished by a human mediator. In circumstances where the opportunities for daily social interaction are limited and documents have to be relied upon to do the work of parsing patients there may be a case for more structured documentation to support these processes. In addition, hospitals could do worse but to consider placements for nurses in the wider ecologies with which they are required to interact as part of the induction of new recruits and their continuing professional development. As we have seen in earlier chapters in this book, the success of nurses' work in articulating trajectories of care hinges on their organisational knowledge of the relevant activities systems in which they work. In those units where the needs of the populations served are diffuse and there is a requirement to engage with a broad and variable number of services then there is a case for more dedicated discharge liaison nurses who can act as the repositories of this information and span the boundaries between services. While many of the discharge liaison nurses underlined the importance of not de-skilling ward-based nurses in relation to planning transfers of care, the complexity and volume of this work creates very real tensions with the immediate demands of caring for acutely ill patients and with current staffing levels is becoming increasingly unsustainable. There is also a case to be made for considering the unintended consequences for transfers of care, of a culture which encourages the proliferation of local artefacts, and how this might be balanced with greater standardisation and a whole systems approach. This added markedly to the volume of work with which nurses had to contend on a daily basis. Not only was much of it unnecessary, it was also dangerous and arguably indirectly added to the challenges of discharge planning because of the effects of multiple documents on the complexity of the medical record. Reluctant as I am to suggest 'another bloody form', internal transfers, in so far as these are unavoidable, may benefit from a simple checklist requiring the unit of origin to summarise pre-specified information necessary to facilitate their work organisation of the new service. While this may not obviate the need for social interaction to support handover, it provides a useful orientating framework to support nurses' sensemaking. There would also be value in developing a daily summary pro forma, so that the current status of individual trajectories encapsulated in nurses' trajectory narratives, was entered into the formal record. As we saw in Chapter 2, this was documented in nurses' handover sheets but discarded at the end of the shift. Not only would this provide a valuable resource for the purposes of creating a working knowledge, but it could also be a short-cut to the information of relevance for the purposes of trajectory crystallisation necessary for transfers of care. It would also go some way to formalising and making visible nurses' responsibilities for trajectory articulation.

Conclusions

In this chapter I have examined the work of nurses in parsing patients for the purposes of transfers of care. I have argued that patients traverse multiple interfaces over an illness episode and that transfers of care represent crystallisation points, at which, through a double translational process, trajectories are stabilised and patient identities reconfigured for the purposes of handover. Artefacts are central to these processes and their completion placed different demands on nurses at different sites within the healthcare system. While certain service boundaries were effectively mediated, elsewhere interface management was more challenging. There is a growing appreciation of the importance of interface management for the quality, safety and efficiency of patient care and yet less recognition of the nature and demands of this work and the time it entails. Nurses were required to fulfil this function in the turbulence of the clinical environment which was subject to constant interruptions and I have no doubt that for a whole range of reasons interface management in certain parts of the organisation was considerably more burdensome and risky than it needed to be. Given the significant contribution nurses make to navigating departmental and organisational interfaces and the fact that parsing patients depends on understanding the work purposes of the transfer destination, nurses would benefit from greater exposure to the wider ecologies with which they interact in order to better fulfil this function. As I have argued in the preceding chapters, activity system knowledge is vital in supporting nurses' organising work, but in order for practitioners to shape the quality of care at service interfaces, broader system understanding is required. With their organisational and clinical knowledge nurses should be well-placed to lead improvement initiatives in this field. But for any of this to happen, it is first necessary to move away from the metaphor of the baton handover to that of parsing patient identities.

Notes

1 George Brown is a distant family member, and sadly passed away later the same year. This extract has been crafted from a comprehensive letter of complaint sent to the hospital in question which catalogues a whole series of shortcomings in George's care. This example is used here with the consent of the family who requested that George should not remain anonymous in the hope that his experiences could be used to address service shortcomings for the benefit of others.
2 I have, however, been funded by The Health Foundation to undertake a study of this kind, as part of the Improvement Science Fellowship which has supported the writing of this book.
3 This is a reference to wound dehiscence, a surgical complication in which a wound ruptures along a surgical incision.

References

Berg, M. (1992). 'The construction of medical disposals: medical sociology and medical problem solving in clinical practice.' *Sociology of Health & Illness* 14(2): 151–180.
Brown, J.S. and P. Duguid (1996). 'The social life of documents.' *First Monday* 1: 1.
Bryan, K., Gage, H. and K. Gilbert (2005). 'Delayed transfer of care of older people from hospital: causes and policy implications.' *Health Policy* 76: 194–201.
Carlile, P.R. (2002). 'A pragmatic view of knowledge and boundaries: boundary objects in new product development.' *Organization Science* 13(4): 442–455.
—— (2004). 'Transferring, translating, and transforming: an integrative framework for managing knowledge across boundaries.' *Organization Science* 15(5): 555–568.
Catchpole, K., de Leval, M.R., McEwan, A., Pigott, N., Elliott, M.J., McQuillan, A., MacDonald, C. and A.J. Goldman (2007). 'Patient handover from surgery to intensive care: using Formula 1 pit-stop and aviation models to improve safety and quality.' *Pediatric Anesthesia* 17: 470–478.
Currie, L. and L. Watterson (2008). *Improving the Safe Transfer of Care: A Quality Improvement Inititive. Final Report.* Oxford, Royal College of Nursing.
Hacking, I. (2004). 'Between Michel Foucault and Erving Goffman: between discourse in the abstract and face-to-face interaction.' *Economy and Society* 33(3): 277–302.
—— (2007). 'Kinds of people: moving targets.' *Proceedings of the British Academy* 151: 285–318.
Kripalani, S., LeFevre, F., Phillips, C.O., Williams, M.V., Basaviah, P. and D.W. Baker (2007). 'Deficits in communication and information transfer between hospital-based and primary care physicians: implications for patient safety and continuity of care.' *JAMA* 297(8): 831–841.
Lee, C. (2007). 'Boundary negotiating artifacts: unbinding the routine of boundary objects and embracing chaos in collaborative work.' *Computer Supported Cooperative Work* (16): 307–339.
Levina, N. and E. Vaast (2005). 'The emergence of boundary spanning competence in practice: implications for implementation and use of information systems.' *MIS Quarterly* 20: 335–363.

National Leadership and Innovation Agency for Healthcare (2008). *Passing the Baton.* Llanharan, Wales, National Leadership and Innovation Agency for Healthcare.

Raban, M.Z. and J. Westbrook (2013). 'Are interventions to reduce interruptions and errors during medication administration effective? A systematic review.' *BMJ Quality & Safety* doi: 10.1136/bmjqs-2013-002118

Scott, J., Williams, D., Ingram, J. and F. Mackenzie (2010). 'The effectiveness of drug round tabards in reducing the incidence of medication errors.' *Nursing Times* 106(34): 13–15.

Strauss, A. (1985). 'Work and the division of labor.' *The Sociological Quarterly* 26(1): 1–19.

6 Rethinking hospital organisation, rethinking nursing

In this book I have examined a little-studied and poorly-understood facet of nursing practice: organising work. My aim has been to bring about a figure-ground reversal and illuminate this largely invisible dimension of the nursing role in order to better understand its content, form and function and uncover the skills and knowledge that underpin it. This is an essential foundational task in order to inform ongoing debates about the contemporary nursing mandate as well as wider efforts to improve service quality. Their location in the sites of care and at critical departmental and organisational interfaces casts nurses in a pivotal role in mediating the relationships between the heterogeneous actors through which patient and population needs are addressed. Through four interrelated domains of practice nurses function as obligatory passage points in hospital orders: creating the working knowledge that supports care delivery; articulating the configurations of socio-material actors required to meet individual needs; matching people with beds and supporting patient flows; and parsing patient identities to secure transfers of care. Not only is this work an essential driver of action, it also operates as a powerful countervailing force to the centrifugal tendencies inherent in healthcare organisations which, for all their gloss of order and rationality, are actually very loose arrangements. In writing about nurses' organising work it has been necessary to write too about these system features: they make this work necessary. This is why, despite including community nurses in the study sample and having wrestled with the writing process for many months, I elected to focus here on hospital nurses. Organising work has different characteristics in different work settings and it was not possible to do justice to the analysis of both community and hospital contexts in a single book. It is also the case that studying everyday practices reveals what social structures look like from within rather than through formal external organisational plans (Anderson and Sharrock 1993) and when viewed from the vantage point of nurses, our understanding of hospital organisation is fundamentally challenged. So not only has it been necessary to write about the healthcare system in order to write about nurses' work, it has also been necessary to write about this differently.

Each of the data chapters of this book has revealed the mismatch between dominant cultural understandings of the rational means through which modern hospitals go about their business and the organisational forms best suited to supporting everyday delivery processes. As well as offering a glimpse of the real-life work behind external appearances this has also involved exposing how prevailing approaches to the challenges of achieving quality, safety and efficiency, often interfere with day-to-day service provision. Thus, in Chapter 2, I questioned orthodox assumptions about the role of the medical record as a mechanism of inter-professional communication in order to make sense of the work of nurses in creating, maintaining and circulating trajectory narratives. I argued that the growing expectation for transparent processes in healthcare has emphasised the archival functions of the medical record at the expense of its value in supporting everyday care delivery. Compensatory systems are therefore required and the work of nurses fulfils this need. In Chapter 3, in examining the nursing contribution to trajectory articulation, I was obliged first to unsettle traditional ideas about multidisciplinary teams. I suggested that far from being a collaborative endeavour in the orthodox sense of this word, patient trajectories might more accurately be understood as comprised of multiple activities and goals, undertaken in parallel and sometimes in opposition, with only brief intersection points where actors come together to align their activities (Munkvold and Ellingsen 2007). While such arrangements make service integration challenging, I have maintained that they are necessary in order for providers to function flexibly in an unpredictable and turbulent system and where the nature of the work is such that it will never be possible to exert the same level of process control as that which can be achieved in industry. Describing nurses' contribution to bed management in Chapter 4, I highlighted the relationship between the evolution of individual patient trajectories and the changing state of the hospital and wider community. Viewed through a nursing lens, it was impossible to conceive of patients and organisational structures as discrete entities. Each has interests which must be negotiated and accommodated. Policy makers misdirect when they present patient 'pathways' as arrangements that are managed for better or for worse within organisations designed for this purpose. In reality they are enfolded into each other as the interests of each are accommodated in the practical delivery of healthcare. These observations are particularly evident in the modifications and adjustments required to secure a match between the needs of patients and the available services. Finally, in Chapter 5, I suggested that transfers of care, generally conceptualised as a matter of role clarity and information exchange, might be understood more accurately as 'parsing work' in which patients are translated from the work object of one service into that of another, transforming individual's identities in the process.

As insights from new institutionalism have shown us, this disconnection between the formal hospital plan and the reality of everyday practice reflects the importance of certain widely accepted cultural models in conferring legitimacy within the field in which organisations function. One of the challenges for nursing, then, is for its own practices to be treated as legitimate. In the first instance this requires a language and knowledge base with which to articulate nursing's distinctive *organising logic* and from which nurses might not only challenge the imposition of culturally dominant, but disruptive, technologies on their work, but also develop new tools to support their practice. In the first part of this final chapter, I will draw together the study findings to consider what these make known about the social organisation of hospital work, the place of nursing within this and how we might conceptualise this relationship. In the second, I will reflect on the overall implications of this study for the future of nursing and healthcare organisation.

The social organisation of hospital work

Throughout this book, I have deployed the notion of care trajectory as a central organising concept, which, because of its roots in the negotiated order perspective, emphasised everyday delivery processes over formal organisational structures. Since its introduction to the literature, the concept of a trajectory has become part of the everyday language of medical sociologists. However, as a framework for analysing the actors and processes associated with patient care it is more limited. This is because, while stressing the linkages within trajectories of care and the 'thick context of organizational possibilities, constraints, and contingencies' in which they are negotiated, Strauss *et al.* (1985) does not provide any basis for analysing these relationships. They provide vivid depictions of patient trajectories – the false starts, blind alleys and changes in direction – but the organisational context, work relationships, tools, technologies and negotiation processes remain hidden from view (Allen *et al.* 2004). As a consequence, the concept does not furnish the analytic resources to understand the relationships between actors and explain why trajectories take the shape that they do. In order to bridge this gap I have taken a practice-based approach and drawn on insights from ANT.

ANT is concerned to 'follow the actors' and hospital work has been considered here from the standpoint of nurses. What emerges from this analysis is an image of health service provision as a stochastic, contingent and distributed process in which patient identities are figured and reconfigured according to the purposes at hand and the organisation is in turn shaped and reshaped by the demands of the populations served. Far from being a managed linear pathway through the service, for much of the time an individual's healthcare is an amorphous network of heterogeneous elements and the patient, as work object, is widely distributed. It is through the work that nurses do in aligning actors and bringing about the necessary translations that mediate these relationships that trajectories are mobilised and, when necessary, stabilised to enable concerted action.

In practice-based approaches to work, boundary object theory (Star and Griesemer 1989) has been applied widely to understand cooperation between different social worlds. In the absence of consensus, boundary objects are able to bridge divisions between groups because they satisfy a range of needs. In recent years a body of literature has emerged that explores how artefacts might function as boundary objects in supporting interprofessional working in healthcare and I have drawn on these insights in earlier chapters (Allen 2009; Mackintosh and Sandall 2010; Cooper 2011). There is, however, an alternative and more radical application of boundary object theory that is useful in enlightening understanding of hospital organisation. In their research on technical projects, Garrety and Badham (2000) distinguish between primary and secondary boundary objects; the former referring to the project itself – the object around which activity is organised – and the latter referring to the physical or abstract entities that enable communication across project collaborators. Applying Garrety and Badham's framework to healthcare, it is the patient that is the primary boundary object around which work is organised (see also, Bloomfield and Vurdubakis 1997; Middleton and Brown 2005). One of the defining features of boundary objects, as conceived by Star and Griesemer (1989), is their interpretative flexibility.

> Boundary objects are objects which are plastic enough to adapt to local needs and the constraints of the several parties employing them, yet robust enough to maintain a common identity across sites. They are weakly structured in common use, and become strongly structured in individual site use. [...] They have different meanings in different social worlds but their structure is common enough to more than one world to make them recognizable, a means of translation. The creation and management of boundary objects is a key process in developing and maintaining coherence across intersecting social worlds.
>
> (Star and Griesemer 1989: 393)

Thus, we might argue that healthcare work is not managed or coordinated around the patient as is conventionally portrayed in the rationalising myths beloved by service managers and policy makers, nor is it a 'negotiated' (Strauss 1964) or 'decoupled' (Meyer and Rowan 1977) order as organisational scholars have claimed. Rather, it is the object of the patient in all its interpretative flexibility that enrols the work of actors into recognisable patterns of action – what service managers call pathways of care – and it is nurses who are central in bringing about the translations through which this is accomplished. This is patient-centred healthcare, but not as this is conventionally understood. It is less a case of services being organised around the needs of the patient, and more a case of the 'patient', by dint of the work that nurses do, holding services together, however fragmented these might be. As Finger *et al.* (1993) have underlined, it is often human mediators who are necessary in making boundary objects act as such and it is clear why nursing is so often referred to as the glue in healthcare systems. Considered in these terms then, rather than trying to create order in healthcare systems through reengineering service pathways which inevitably create new disorder in their wake (Berg 1998), we might instead focus on the question of how organisational processes and technologies might strengthen the position of 'patients' in the ordering of their care.

From organising work to organising logic

Throughout this book I have argued that nursing can be considered an obligatory passage point in healthcare organisation. Obligatory passage points are a functional necessity in actor networks and the primary actor through which all others must pass. Nurses are the network builders and principal mediators through which the diverse elements that comprise trajectories of care are aligned and where necessary kept apart. There is very little that moves in healthcare without passing through the hands of a nurse. But if this element of the nursing role is to be taken seriously and nursing is to gain legitimacy for the logic that underpins its organising practice, then it is important to move beyond metaphors and analogies – oil, glue, connective tissue – and develop a formal language through which to describe its mechanisms of action.

Taken as a whole, I suggest that nurses' organising work rests on a constellation of practices that might be termed 'translational mobilisation'. As outlined in Chapter 1, in ANT translation has a dual meaning and both apply here. The semiotic sense of the word encapsulates the work that nurses do at the gateways into the service to transform people and their problems into patients with organisationally recognisable identities, their work in clinical locales in converting trajectory narratives into formats that align with the information needs of providers, their work in parsing patient identities for the purposes of transfers of care at critical interfaces, their work in matching patterns of clinical signs with the appropriate organisational response, their work in integrating trajectory activities so that these do not interfere with each other, and their work in reconciling the needs of patients with available resources. Translation also refers to the movement of an entity in space and time, and so alludes to the role of nurses in managing patient flows, ensuring temporal articulation, and aligning the socio-material configurations that support action. I have combined translation with the notion of mobilisation in preference to that of coordination because organising work extends far beyond aligning and integrating activity. As we have seen, nurses initiate and ensure actions happen in the first place and also develop and implement strategies to overcome obstacles to progress. Furthermore, coordination has connotations of formal processes designed to align conduct according to a pre-defined plan, whereas much of the work that nurses do is in reaction to unexpected contingencies, whether these are clinical or organisational in origin. Mobilisation is also intended to convey something of the energy entailed by organising work and its involved and continuous character.

In shining a light on organising work, one of the aims of the study was to uncover the knowledge and skills that underpin it. The intention was to inform thinking about the nursing mandate and in particular debates about non-nursing duties and also, if indicated, to consider the implications of this for nurse education and professional development. In studying practices ethnographically, one does not search for knowledge in participants' minds in so far as they might talk about it, rather it is located in activities, events and procedures (Mol 2002); and when we scrutinise nurses' organising work it becomes clear that translational mobilisation depends for its success on a combination of clinical and organisational knowledge. That nurses operate with a clinical gaze (Foucault 1973) is well understood (Benner 1984; May 1992), but my data also highlight the importance of organisational awareness too, and it is the synthesis of these two knowledge types that characterises nurses' distinct professional vision (Goodwin 1995). Nurses displayed a detailed understanding of the relevant activity systems in the local ecologies in which they worked, including role formats, routines, bed economy, material and psychological artefacts and temporal structures. This enabled them to locate, accumulate, interpret and make sense of an array of fragmented information sources to create and sustain an ongoing awareness of individual patient trajectories and to combine this with their understanding of organisational structures and routines to make the translations necessary for healthcare delivery. As I argued in Chapter 2, this is clearly a holistic approach to healthcare, and a unique orientation not shared by members of other professional groups. It is, however, a quite different understanding of holism from the bio-psycho-social model that has dominated nursing's public jurisdictional claims in recent history and it is underpinned by a subtly different knowledge base and skill set.

Thus, I have argued that routines featured prominently in nurses' translational mobilisation practices. Much contested within the profession, in the 1980s when nurse academics were pursuing an individualised patient care agenda, associated as they were with hierarchy and task allocation, routines were widely denounced. With the rise of evidence-based practice, routines were again debated but now gilded with the patina of science, they have been accorded greater credibility and more readily, if not altogether uncritically, embraced by the profession (Traynor 2009). In both cases, arguments about routines reflect the tension between professional and managerial logics in the healthcare field and turn on their role in mediating the relationship between nurses and patients: they either protect against the idiosyncratic interventions of individual practitioners or they result in cookbook medicine and depersonalised care. Here, however, I am making a rather different argument. Considered in terms of nurses' organising logic, my data indicate that the value of routines or standards for the purposes of translational mobilisation lies not in their application or rejection in the case of individual patients, but in the role that they play as part of the sensemaking and sensegiving resources (Maitlis and Lawrence 2007) through which trajectories are mobilised. In organisational studies, the importance of routines in supporting decision-making has long been recognised (Cyert and

March 1963). Weick (1979) suggests that routines can be thought of as a 'set of recipes' for connecting episodes of social interaction in an orderly manner and Pentland and Reuter (1994) have likened them to a grammar of organising. This process and practice-based conceptualisation is a rather different understanding of routines from that which has hitherto underpinned debates within the profession.[1]

Translational mobilisation depends too on perspective-taking and an understanding of the needs of organisational members so that information and actions can be converted into terms that are relevant and understandable. This requires sensitivity to the work purposes and concerns of others and an ability to express these in their language. In psychology there is considerable evidence that people find this difficult (Heath and Staudenmayer 2000) and these challenges are all the more exacting in organisations where teams are ephemeral so that staff cannot depend on prior relationships to facilitate understanding, and when communication is not face-to-face but mediated through alternative formats. As we have seen, perspective-taking became increasingly difficult when nurses were required to work with distant personnel whose work processes they were unfamiliar with and when opportunities for direct social interaction were limited.

Translation mobilisation also requires nurses to operate at the interface between individual patients and the organisation and the decisions that are taken in mediating this relationship shape the quality of patient care in important ways. As I have argued, a necessary element of this aspect of nurses' practice was the application of categories through which individual identities were effaced in order to accomplish organising work. Yet while psychological artefacts are useful resources in making sense of a complex field, they always privilege one viewpoint and silence others and it is easy to see how real people and their particular concerns can get lost in these processes. This has particular salience in the context of growing concern for care and compassion and thus central to translational mobilisation is the need for nurses to resist becoming enrolled in managerial logics which privilege efficiency or professional logics which foreground the needs of certain individuals and work to mediate these agenda in the most ethical and humane way possible. As Chambliss (1997) has observed, moral feelings and daily actions are not separate entities and a whole host of moral assumptions are embedded in habitual modes of behaviour.

Finally, in hospital contexts translation mobilisation requires that individuals are able to operate in a turbulent and unpredictable environment. In their classic socio-technical systems study of coal mining, Emery and Trist (1965) distinguished between the production process and the work environment. They classified the latter according to its degree of complexity and developed a typology ranging from the placid randomised environment to that of the 'turbulent field'. According to these authors, the turbulent environment is unstable and is liable to disturbance and demands a particular form of work organisation in order that production may continue. They argue that in coal mining face workers all share a common ability to contend with the underground environment and this is of a higher order skill than the specific operations belonging to the production cycle. Melia (1979) has applied Emery and Trist's notion of the turbulent field to healthcare, and has argued that all nurses require the skills to work in such environments. While I would not propose that the ability to handle the hospital work environment is a higher order skill than that involved in translational mobilisation, it was clear that in the study site the pressures were such that not all nurses were equally able to cope with its demands. For example, in the Emergency Unit a number of individuals – nurses and paramedics – volunteered that they knew the kind of shift they had in store simply by looking at who was designated coordinator for the shift. So, contra Melia, it would appear that not all nurses have this skill, or at least not at the level required in some of the most profoundly tumultuous environments in today's healthcare settings. Indeed, this environmental factor is an important difference between organising work in community and acute care contexts and a possible influence on nurses' career choices. It may also have implications for the ease with which it is possible to combine this element of the nursing function with clinical work within the hospital environment as well as the feasibility of different modes of work organisation.

Overall then, translational mobilisation depends for its success on the synthesis of clinical and organisational knowledge and a professional vision that enables nurses to zoom in and out from the individual to the many and to do so with sufficient intellectual agility, pragmatism and focus, to be able to work flexibly in response to contingencies while at the same time ensuring the progression of planned activity. It depends too on a particular habitus in which organising work activities are interleaved, woven through the fabric of everyday practice with much of the work performed on the fly. In the light of this skill-set and given its involved and continuous nature, it is difficult to see how this function could readily be undertaken by any other occupational group and this may explain the persistence of organising work in the nursing role historically.

Evetts (2011) has suggested that with the growth of neoliberal logics in the private and public sector, a new model of 'organisational professionalism' has emerged alongside the more traditional model, which she terms 'occupational professionalism'. The former, she argues, is oriented to organisational concerns and incorporates rational–legal forms of decision-making, standardisation of work practices, and performance review, whereas the latter is underpinned by trusting relationships with clients and informed by practitioner autonomy and moral codes. According to Evetts these two forms compete with each other. The nurses studied here, actively managed these logics, and on a daily basis accomplished a multitude of accommodations such that these could be reconciled. Everyday nursing practice might better be understood, then, as a hybrid form of professionalism, which combines aspects of Evetts' types but, more importantly, derives its value from the work that is done in mediating the relationship between the different institutional logics these embody. Indeed, rather than these being understood as competing models or contradictory logics, we might think of the potential afforded for knowledge generation by working at their interface.

Back to the future

So where does translational mobilisation take us? Are these just fancy words for what nurses already know as was suggested by one conference delegate when I first presented this work? And at one level of course, the answer to this question is yes. If nurses did not recognise their practice in the descriptions offered here, then that would be cause for concern. At another level, however, while they may acknowledge their work when it is reflected back to them, nurses find it extraordinarily difficult to describe this element of their role, either to themselves or wider society. They are also deeply ambivalent about its value. This is because, although nursing is an organisationally embedded occupation, over the last 40 years it has tended to understand itself through the lens of a prototypical profession predicated on an untrammelled one-to-one relationship with clients. The latter is a poor fit with the reality of everyday nursing practice, however. On the one hand, the constraints of the workplace have encouraged a division of labour in which nurses have largely divested themselves of hands-on care, but are increasingly being called to account for its quality amidst accusations that practitioners are too posh to wash. On the other hand, it fails to capture the breadth of nursing work or the expertise on which this is based. Not only does this generate strains with clinicians' identities, it undermines much of the work that nurses do and discourages any professionally-led efforts to better understand and augment a significant dimension of nursing practice. A corollary of this is that nurses often find themselves having to accommodate technologies that hinder rather than support their work and they are unable to justify their endeavours when these are called into question.

Nurses may aspire to undertake all aspects of patient care, but the economic realities of health services have always made it necessary to modify these professional ideals in response to the material constraints of the work setting. In the main, the fault lines have tended to occur at the boundary between body work, which has increasingly become the responsibility of healthcare assistants (Cavendish 2013), and advanced clinical interventions, care-planning and coordination, undertaken by qualified nurses for those patients for whom they are responsible. But there is evidence that these already attenuated models of practice are currently under considerable strain and in certain environments it is becoming increasingly difficult for nurses to combine organising work with clinical care. There are reports in the literature that certain activities, such as venepuncture, recently delegated from doctors to nurses, are being passed on to healthcare support workers (Cavendish 2013) and at Parklands, while several of the nurse specialist roles combined clinical and organising components, at ward level during core hours these activities were increasingly separated, with the bulk of organising work undertaken by a dedicated shift coordinator who did not carry a clinical caseload. On the one hand, by assuming this responsibility, the shift coordinator functioned as a buffer between patient care and the turbulence of the organisation which was positively valued. As we have seen, personnel from outside the clinical areas appreciated having a single point of contact and nurses caring for patients clinically could undertake this work uninterrupted. On the other hand, in most of the areas I studied, the coordinator role was performed by the senior nurse on duty and this often left relatively inexperienced nurses and healthcare assistants responsible for direct patient care. This made supervision of clinical practice challenging, and also created concerns about the professional development of junior nurses considered to be in danger of becoming deskilled.[2] There are very real risks, then, that left unchecked, the requirement to cope with the daily demands of hospital work will continue to pull apart the clinical and organisational knowledge bases on which nursing work depends.

Nursing work has been portrayed here against the backdrop of burgeoning administrative loads which undoubtedly make organising work more onerous. A survey published by the Royal College of Nursing estimated that nurses spend 2.5 million hours a week on purportedly non-essential paperwork, which equates to 17.3 per cent of all hours worked by NHS nurses in the UK (RCN 2013). In the context of growing concern about the demands made on frontline staff by unnecessary bureaucracy and, following the Francis Inquiry (House of Commons 2013), in England the NHS Confederation undertook a government commissioned review of 'paperwork' (NHS Confederation 2013). The subsequent report made recommendations for reducing the bureaucratic burden placed on providers by national bodies, which they estimated was responsible for 25 per cent of the load, and they urged a similar review of local bodies, believed to be responsible for an additional 25 per cent. Little is said, however, about healthcare organisations themselves, attributed in the report with 45 per cent of the administrative freight, and which at Parklands, clearly contributed to nurses' workloads and for which, somewhat ironically, nurses themselves were partly responsible.

In recent years nursing has emerged as the lead profession in quality improvement initiatives and nurses have been charged with the development and implementation of a range of artefacts, technologies and interventions which purport to augment service processes (Allen 2009, 2010a, b, 2014). Given their unacknowledged organising work function, such approaches have a self-evident appeal as a means through which nurses can both draw on their systems understanding and render this visible. Moreover, when behaviour cannot be coerced through direct orders, standards and technologies can help fill the gap to coordinate activity (Brunsson and Jacobsson 2000) and as we have seen, nurses have uncertain authority in performing this element of their role. It is also the case that while nursing tasks are increasingly devolved to healthcare assistants, supervision is becoming increasingly difficult and there is a growing trend to look to non-human actors to fulfil this function (Allen 2014). For example, at the time of the study, Parklands, like many modern health services, was introducing an Early Warning Scoring System for the purposes of recording patient observations. This entailed colour coded domains on the vital signs recording chart which signalled the need for senior review. The system has been introduced in response to growing concerns about patient mortality and morbidity arising from a 'failure to rescue' that is, not intervening in a timely manner when vital signs indicate that a patient's condition is deteriorating. Similar observations might also be made about 'intentional rounding', a quality intervention in the form of a checklist designed to ensure attention is paid to patients' comfort, pressure area care and hydration, and which generates a record that this has occurred, which was also being implemented in the study site.

Yet while there is some evidence to indicate that protocols can have an empowering effect on nursing staff (Mackintosh and Sandall 2010), it is less clear how far these technologies function in an unmediated way to safeguard services (Allen 2012, 2014). As we have seen, to some extent their proliferation reflects dominant beliefs about the appropriate organisational response to widespread concerns about the quality and safety of health services and there are some who have argued for the need to take a 'reality check' on checklists (Bosk *et al.* 2009). In the context of increasingly stretched frontline services it is easy to see the seductive power of the laminated promises of improvement tools for nursing staff, but the volume and complexity of the technologies generated in the interests of service quality often confound the very processes they are designed to improve and may increase the attendant administrative work. It may be an uncomfortable fact therefore that in order to exert greater control over their work, unwittingly, nurses may be contributing to the very burdens about which they themselves complain.

Since it was developed in the nineteenth century, nursing has always included an organisational component. Traditional readings of nursing history have described the struggle for and against nurse registration in terms of the tension between Nightingale's vocational model of nursing, based on good moral character and on the job training, and the professional model advocated by Mrs Bedford Fenwick based on private practice, which emphasised technical and scientific skills. But as Gamarnikow (1984, 1991) has argued, this overlooks the fact that what was at issue were contested definitions of nursing rather than the position of nursing within the overall healthcare division of labour and central to this was nursing's relationship with medicine. Thus while the two sides argued over the class and requirements of recruits to the profession, the basic model of nursing they proposed was very similar. Reformers were heavily influenced by the proto feminist theory of Jameson that there were natural spheres of activity for men and women which was believed to be rooted in the family. Thus work outside the home ought to resemble work in the home. The model of nursing that emerged was based on the organisation of domestic work in the middle class Victorian household and was designed to discipline both nurses and hospitals, problems of supervision and coordination familiar to middle class women as domestic managers. For example, contrary to popular folklore, in her first appointment as superintendent, Florence Nightingale '[w]as not the deliverer of care, but the organizer of other's labour' and '[h]er improvements had as much to do with increasing the productivity of the staff and enhancing the sanitary conditions as with directly improving the comfort of patients' (Dingwall *et al.* 1988: 40).

The social position occupied by the matron in the hospital power structure also resembled that she would have occupied in the home (Carpenter 1977): the matron became the symbolic wife of the consultant and established a separate sphere of autonomy in her managerial control of those under her. A good deal of medical resistance to nursing registration was grounded in the fear that the organisational independence of nursing could make them a potential source of quasi-medical practitioner. The idea gradually gained strength that cure and care processes were separate from each other (Carpenter 1977). Thus by making its case for a distinctive profession for women based on care, nurses' practice was dependent on the medical profession in designating the patient qua patient which served to counter any concerns about the threat nursing posed to the position of medicine and to allay any concerns that nurses (women) would be organising the work of men (doctors), even if that was what they were doing in fact.

At different times over its occupational history it has been unclear whether nursing's progress should be through absorbing medically devolved tasks, strengthening its administrative functions (Carpenter 1977) or the pursuit of autonomous status. Over the last 40 years, however, driven in part by the influence of North American academic nurses, oriented to a trait model of professionalism,[3] and desirous of establishing a domain of autonomous practice with an underpinning independent professional knowledge base, patient care has emerged at the heart of the profession's claim to specialist expertise. It is also the case that appeals to 'care' furnished nursing with an indefeasible argument with which to advance the interests of the profession; after all who could be against 'care'? In reality, however, as I have argued, these aspirations have always been broken on the wheel of nursing's licence and organising work has continued to remain an important aspect of everyday practice. To reinstate organising work into the contemporary mandate, then, is not a departure from modern day nursing's foundations nor is it a derogation of nursing knowledge and skills. Indeed, given the complexity of today's healthcare systems, to reformulate the nursing mandate more inclusively to include nurses' contribution to the organisation of healthcare underlines the importance of graduate level nurses because of the sophisticated technical, supervisory, organisational and social skills necessary to undertake this work.

While nursing may always have had an organisational component, its content, form and function in contemporary healthcare systems has singular features arising from a specific historical context which have greatly increased the demands of this work. Patients admitted to hospital are more acutely ill than once they were and many are frail, elderly and have co-morbidities, magnifying the challenges of trajectory articulation. Specialisation, coupled with accelerated patient throughput, has increased the work involved in transfers of care and bed management creating a continuous 'churn' (Duffield *et al.* 2007) with which nurses must contend. Pressure on resources has made it progressively more difficult to secure discharge from hospital and because patients move through the system more quickly, activity that in the past could be extended over several days is compressed into ever decreasing time-frames (Duffield *et al.* 2007). All of this has taken place against the backdrop of wider changes to the workforce which has seen an overall reduction in qualified nurses (Ball *et al.* 2013), a concomitant growth in healthcare assistants and a rebalancing of specialist and generalist nursing skill mix and spiralling demands on frontline staff for paperwork and data entry (Royal College of Nursing 2013; Cavendish 2013; NHS Confederation 2013).

Throughout this book I have argued that organising work is enormously important for the quality of patient care and the efficiency of healthcare systems and that nurses' occupational niche and unique skill set makes them logical candidates to fulfil this function. But for a whole range of reasons this aspect of the role is undoubtedly more challenging than it needs to be and coping with its demands within current staffing levels and skill mix creates an impetus towards models of practice which, in the longer term, threaten to pull apart the clinical and organisational knowledge on which the work depends. Its demands also make it increasingly difficult to supervise the work of healthcare assistants and inexperienced nurses. It is unsurprising, then, that as the volume and complexity of organising work has grown, nurses have been so readily attracted to technologies that either purport to reduce its burdens or offer the promise of safeguarding standards of care (Allen 2014). A mandate based exclusively on nurses' care-giving functions is clearly unsustainable within such a context and there are unmistakable indications that service quality is suffering. While the content of contemporary nursing work is shaped by the intersection of complex demographic, economic and technological forces, the point I want to press here is of the consequences for nursing and for society of continued institutionalised ignorance of nurses' organising work. The challenge for the profession is first to recognise its own practices as legitimate and second, to ensure significant others treat these as such.

A brave new world?

In the final section of this book, I want to envisage an alternative future, in which organising work is reinstated in the contemporary nursing mandate, nurses are equipped with a vocabulary with which to articulate their practice, translational mobilisation is taken seriously, and healthcare is informed by nurses' organising logic. What could such a brave new world look like?

Firstly, organising work would be factored into workload models. There is growing international concern about nurse staffing levels and an accumulative body of evidence that points to the relationship between skill mix and the quality and safety of patient care. The use of a higher proportion of registered nurses is associated with better health outcomes, shorter lengths of stay and reduced patient morbidity (Aiken *et al.* 2012; Jacob *et al.* 2013). Within the UK there is huge variation in both nursing numbers and skill mix (Audit Commission 2001; Ball *et al.* 2013). Staff shortages were implicated in the unacceptable quality of care reported at Mid Staffordshire NHS Trust leading to calls from the profession for the establishment of mandatory minimum nurse-to-patient ratios, like those in place in California (Aiken *et al.* 2010). This has been thus far resisted, but from April 2014 in England trusts will be expected to publish their nurse staffing levels monthly on a national patient safety website and there is an expectation that recommendations will be made on indicative nurse-to-patient ratios in different settings. Yet although a considerable amount of effort has been invested in developing workforce models over the last 40 years, questions remain as to their overall utility and relevance to health service provision. Indeed, there is no established staffing or skill mix model that addresses all the variables that impact on nurses' workload (Flynn and McKeown 2009), unsurprising, perhaps, given that much of nursing work is poorly understood. Furthermore, models for determining skill mix tend, on the whole, to be predicated on clinical rather than organisational factors and are overdetermined by considerations of patient acuity. This reflects the prevailing view of nursing practice as primarily about advanced direct patient care, such that in those clinical areas where patients require mainly support with activities of daily living rather than technical interventions, the number of qualified staff is rather lower. Yet as we have seen, the work of nurses is shaped to a considerable extent by the translational mobilisation burdens in the locales in which they practice. One of the potential impacts of this study is that it lays the ground for the development of formal measures of the demands of organising work in clinical care areas – such as the complexity of health and social care needs of the populations served, the throughput of patients, the variety of unfamiliar organisations and departments with which the unit is required to work – which could be built into workload models. Furthermore, it might also throw into sharp relief those aspects of the system that are unduly burdensome and where process improvement is indicated.

Translation mobilisation depends to a considerable extent on nurses' understanding of local activity systems. Future models of nursing practice would take into account the optimal content and scope of the knowledge necessary to enable nurses to realise their potential within the service ecologies in which they work. As we have seen, when nurses were required to practice beyond the boundaries of their local context, such as in those cases where transfers of care had to be accomplished with services with which they were unfamiliar, then translational mobilisation became more challenging. The limits of this knowledge, and the challenges of localisation for organising work, helps to explain too, nurses' reluctance to be redeployed in areas that they did not know. Translational mobilisation processes might be augmented by arranging nursing work so that clinicians have opportunities to broaden their understanding of the systems with which they are required to interact, through formal induction processes, service rotations or secondments. This may also afford greater flexibility for staff to be deployed where they are needed in response to the vicissitudes of the workplace without being deskilled by the process. These considerations are relevant to quality initiatives too. Localisation is a core tenet of contemporary improvement models; it is believed to foster grassroots ownership. In a future in which translational mobilisation was taken seriously the boundaries of clinical micro systems for the purposes of quality improvement would be reviewed and pertinent questions asked about the most appropriate level and scale at which to intervene in the organisation.

Most of the nurses I shadowed were experienced and had spent many years working within the organisation. Their translational mobilisation skills were not plug and play capacities, but had been developed and built up over time and were integrated with the surroundings. My observations on the gastro-intestinal surgical ward revealed this very clearly. The unit had recently relocated from another hospital within the Health Board and at the time of the fieldwork the senior nurses were struggling to navigate the organisational structures in the new site. Similarly, the intensive care services had been reorganised and nurses, who in the past had only ever worked in one satellite facility, were now required to work in the main hospital. For all their experience, they did not have familiarity with the local systems and processes necessary to assume the shift coordinator role, which had important implications for planning staff rosters. This raises interesting questions about how these limitations can be overcome. A reinstatement of organising work into the core nursing function would necessitate the development of new models of nurse education and professional development so that the knowledge and skills that underpin translational mobilisation could be taught. It might also include thinking imaginatively about how the understanding on which organising work rests might be made more widely available, to enable this to be more readily shared. This is a necessary prerequisite to facilitate practice models in which clinical and organising work can be more closely coupled and staff are not deskilled when they move to different parts of the organisation. New information systems clearly have a role here. A future in which organising work was taken seriously would see investment in technologies that make available the organisational information necessary to support translational mobilisation. This might include central information on services, referral and transfer processes, and routines and protocols, all electronically available in a handheld device or smart phone, such that they can be easily accessed. They would be of particular value in supporting nurses caring for outlying patients or who are unfamiliar with the unit and junior nurses too, who are perhaps less au fait with their local clinical micro system. Moreover, they would better facilitate the involvement of patients and their families in the planning process. At present, contemporary information systems make this very difficult. In the past, new technologies have often proved disappointing to clinicians as these have tended to be developed to support archival functions rather than frontline work processes. In our brave new world nurses would be fully engaged with development processes and able to articulate their practice so that these logics are built into the design of systems and technologies.

While wider exposure can broaden one's organisational knowledge and systems awareness, and information technologies might be developed to make organisational knowledge more extensively available, translational mobilisation still requires this to be synthesised with clinical knowledge. At Parklands, much of this sensemaking was made visible through nursing handover through the circulation of trajectory narratives and these learning opportunities are at risk of being lost by recent quality improvement efforts that endeavour to make nursing handover more efficient. Yet as Nonaka and Takeuchi (1995) have argued, there is value in sharing information with people who do not immediately need it. Rather than being a source of organisation inefficiency, redundancy can be an important mechanism for learning and in particular the transmission of tacit knowledge. Nonaka and Takeuchi refer to this as 'learning by intrusion'. To take translational mobilisation seriously, then, is to better understand how these skills are acquired in practice.

In our brave new world, nurses' organising role would have official recognition. At Parklands, in a number of locales certain nurses were emerging as the lead professional in coordinating complex care arrangements and appeared to be accorded the local power to successfully fulfil this function. But these arrangements were aligned with organisational priorities around discharge planning rather than nurses' generic organising role function and the extent to which role incumbents' commanded authority appeared to reflect the idiosyncrasies of the individuals concerned and the different clinical micro systems in which they operated rather than this being formally mandated. If we were to take translational mobilisation seriously, in the future nurses' organising role would be formally recognised and nurses would have the authority to make things happen. Healthcare organisation would also confer upon others, including doctors, the obligation to orient their own practices to such arrangements.

Nurses are increasingly taking leading roles in quality improvement, and given their activity system knowledge and understanding of the clinical–organisational interface they are well-placed to progress this work. Indeed, ethnographic study of their practice reveals a deep understanding of local organisational processes, and a more sophisticated understanding of improvement technologies than they are often given credit for, or at least by social scientists (Allen 2009). Yet the evidence suggests that they are often poorly supported in these roles (Allen 2014) and, unable to communicate what they know, they may be seduced by healthcare's rationalising myths and are guilty of embracing new technologies uncritically and applying them in ways or in contexts which limit their effectiveness or have unintended negative consequences. In a brave new world in which translational mobilisation was taken seriously, nurses would be using their organising knowledge and understanding to have a leading role in improving service quality, but engaging with these processes in more confident and sophisticated ways. Safety and quality improvement methodology is increasingly being incorporated into pre- and post-registration curricula of all health professionals. At present limited to a 'tools and techniques' approach, there is a growing recognition of the need for more critical understanding of these issues, at least for those senior clinicians and managers who are increasingly required to lead developments in this field.

Conclusion

Although nursing work has always had an organising component, in recent history this has tended to be regarded as the dirty work of the profession and a distraction from nurses' 'real work' with patients. In this book, through the detailed scrutiny of the everyday practices of nurses in a large UK NHS Health Board, I have cast patient care into shadow to illuminate the nursing contribution to everyday service delivery. I have argued that unremarkable as it first appears, nurses' organising work contributes in important ways to the quality, safety and efficiency of healthcare and that recognising its content, form and function and the knowledge, skills and logic that underpin it has important implications for our efforts to improve the service. Understanding organising work helps us to comprehend why quality improvement initiatives founder or have unintended negative consequences on service delivery because these do not take into account pre-existing work processes. Indeed, when healthcare systems are viewed through the lens of nurses' organising practices, they take on a rather different hue from that assumed by orthodox perspectives. Healthcare is not managed or coordinated around the patient as is conventionally assumed, nor is it simply a 'negotiated' (Strauss 1964) or 'decoupled' (Meyer and Rowan 1977) order; rather, it is the patient as boundary object that enrols the work of actors into recognisable patterns of action and it is nurses who as obligatory passage points in the network bring about the translations through which this is accomplished.

I have suggested that the mechanisms by which nurses have this effect can be understood as a process of translational mobilisation which depends for its success on the synthesis of clinical and organisational knowledge, a professional vision capable of zooming in and out from the individual to the many and the ability to make sense of and create order in a fast-flowing turbulent environment. This skill set and the fact that translational mobilisation is continuous and involved with the sites of care, suggests that nurses continue to be best placed to fulfil this function. Nevertheless, my data suggest that the demands of organising work in contemporary healthcare systems are such that it is increasingly difficult for this to be combined with the clinical element of the nursing role, which threatens to disengage the knowledge bases on which translational mobilisation depends. Because nursing struggles to recognise its own practices as legitimate and have others treat these as such, organising work is undoubtedly more onerous than it needs to be, and I have sketched out a future vision of practice, in which nurses' organising logic is taken seriously and organising work is reinstated into the nursing mandate.

Healthcare services across high-income countries face considerable pressures to improve the safety, quality and efficiency of their processes in a context of significant financial constraint and changes in the demographic profiles of the populations served. In the UK, these tensions had come to a head at precisely the point this book was being written. Reports appeared in the media almost daily about the pressures on services, with calls from many constituencies for fundamental changes to the current system (Future Hospital Commission 2013), the instigation of several government commissioned reviews (Clwyd and Hart 2013; NHS Confederation 2013), as well as professionally-driven papers (Future Hospital Commission 2013) and academic policy analyses (Ham *et al.* 2012; Imison and Bohmer 2013); all set against the backdrop of considerable public disquiet about the quality of fundamental care standards and a sense that in some sectors, staffs have lost their compassion to care. Unless translational mobilisation is taken seriously there are very real risks that as service managers respond to the overwhelming pressures that confront the service, this could make organising work and patient care all the more challenging.

The world of work is constantly changing and the analysis presented here must be understood as a historical snapshot at a particular time and in a particular place. It is also the case that organising work is intimately bound up with the contexts in which it is located and more research is needed to better understand how this element of the nursing role is shaped by different locales. For reasons already outlined, the scope of this study was restricted to adult care nurses working in the hospital context and how far the findings represented here arise from singular features of the work setting in which the research was undertaken is uncertain. Further inquiries will be beneficial to identify similarities and differences across different fields of practice and different organisational, national and regional contexts. My hope is that this study has laid the foundations for further work and that it offers a useful framework through which to think more systematically about this element of the nursing role and which might be extended and developed further through new applications.

And finally...

There is a widely held view that all systems tend towards disorder and that energy is required to maintain order. Nurses are the source of this energy in healthcare. Formal organisations have a tendency to overestimate their orderliness and the degree to which their activities are governed by rational systems and processes. Yet in so far as healthcare exhibits any order, the findings of this study show, this must be understood as a nursing order.

Notes

1 Bloor (1976) has challenged the predominant cognitive understanding of decision-making, suggesting that medical decision-making is tied to routine practices and individual decision rules.

2 In the community, too, coordinator roles were also emerging in response to the growing number of vulnerable people living with complex chronic conditions considered to be at high risk of an unnecessary hospital admission. Beyond the immediate research site, in the community mental health nursing context, Simpson (2005) has argued that the demands of care coordination are squeezing out the clinical aspects of the nursing role and on the other side of the Atlantic, in the North American context, Gittell and Weiss (2004) observe in passing that owing to the acceleration of patient throughput and reduced length of stay, coordination is no longer possible for the primary care nurse and that increasingly this responsibility is being placed in the hands of – non-nurse – case managers.

3 This involved drawing up a list of criteria of a profession by which various occupations could be matched. Relevant traits included: possession and use of expert or specialist knowledge, exercise of autonomous thought and judgement and responsibility to wider society through voluntaristic commitment to a set of principles (Hoyle and John 1995). While the approach has been largely discredited in social science, it has nevertheless acted as a useful reference point on which occupations aspiring to professional status have sought to strengthen their social standing.

References

Aiken, L.H., Sloane, D.M. and H.L. Smith (2010). 'Implications of the California nurse staffing mandate for other states.' *Health Services Research* 45(4): 904–921.

Aiken, L.H., Sermeus, W., Van den Heed, K., Sloane, D.M., Busse, R., McKee, M., Bruyneel, L., Rafferty, A.M., Griffiths, P., Moreno-Casbas, M.T., Tishelman, C., Scott, A., Brzostek, T., Kinnunen, J., Schwendimann, E., Heinen, M., Zikos, D., Sjetne, I.S., Smith, H.L. and A. Kutney-Lee (2012). 'Patient safety, satisfaction, and quality of hospital care: cross sectional surveys of nurses and patients in 12 countries in Europe and the United States.' *BMJ* 344(1717): 1–14.

Allen, D. (2009). 'From boundary concept to boundary object: the politics and practices of care pathway development.' *Social Science & Medicine* 69: 354–361.

—— (2010a). 'Care pathways: an ethnographic description of the field.' *International Journal of Care Pathways* 14: 47–51.

—— (2010b). 'Care pathways: some social scientific observations on the field.' *International Journal of Care Pathways* 14: 4–9.

—— (2012). 'Situated context for quality improvement purposes: artefacts, affordances and socio-technical infrastructure.' *Health: An Interdisciplinary Journal for the Social Study of Health, Illness and Medicine* 17 (5): 460–477.

—— (2014). 'Lost in translation? "Evidence" and the articulation of institutional logics in integrated care pathways: from positive to negative boundary object?' *Sociology of Health & Illness.*

Allen, D., Griffiths, L. and P. Lyne (2004). 'Understanding complex trajectories in health and social care provision.' *Sociology of Health & Illness* 26(7): 1008–1030.

Anderson, R. and W. Sharrock (1993). 'Can organizations afford knowledge?' *Computer Supported Cooperative Work* 1: 143–162.

Audit Commission (2001). *Acute Hospitals Portfolio Review of National Findings: Ward Staffing.* London, The Stationery Office.

Ball, J.E., Murrells, T., Rafferty, A.M., Morrow, E. and P. Griffiths (2013). '"Care left undone" during nursing shifts: associations with workload and perceived quality of care.' *BMJ Quality and Safety.* Published Online First DOI: 10.1136/bjmjqs-2012-001767.

Benner, P. (1984). *From Novice to Expert, Excellence and Power in Clinical Nursing Practice.* Menlo Park, CA, Addison-Wesley Publishing Company.

Berg, M. (1998). Order(s) and disorder(s): of protocols and medical practices. *Differences in Medicine: Unravelling Practices, Techniques, and Bodies.* M. Berg and A. Mol. Durham and London, Duke University Press: 226–246.

Bloomfield, B. and T. Vurdubakis (1997). Paper traces: inscribing organizations and information technology. *Information Technology and Organizations: Strategies, Networks and Integration.* B. Bloomfield, R. Coombs, D. Knights and D. Littler. Oxford, Oxford University Press: 85–112.

Bloor, M. (1976). 'Bishop Berkeley and the adenotonsillectomy enigma: an exploration of variation in the construction of medical disposals.' *Sociology* 10(1): 43–61.

Bosk, C.L., Dixon-Woods, M., Goeschel, C. and P. Pronovost (2009). 'Reality check for check lists.' *The Lancet* 374(9688): 444–445.

Brunsson, N. and B. Jacobsson, Eds. (2000). *A World of Standards.* Oxford, Oxford University Press.

Carpenter, M. (1977). The new managerialism and professionalism in nursing. *Health and the Division of Labour.* M. Stacey, M. Reid, C. Heath and R. Dingwall. London, Croom Helm.

Cavendish, C. (2013). The Cavendish Review: An Independent Review into Healthcare Assistants and Support Workers in the NHS and Social Care Settings.

Chambliss, D. (1997). *Beyond Caring: Hospitals, Nurses, and the Social Organization of Ethics.* Chicago, University of Chicago Press.

Clwyd, A. and T. Hart (2013). *NHS Hospital Complaints System Review: Putting Patients Back in the Picture.* London, Department of Health.

Cooper, R.J. (2011). 'In praise of the prescription: the symbolic and boundary object value of the traditional prescription in the electronic age.' *Health Sociology Review* 20(4): 462–474.

Cyert, R.M. and J.G. March (1963). *A Behavioral Theory of the Firm.* Englewood Cliffs, NJ, Prentice-Hall.

Dingwall, R., Rafferty, A.M and C. Webster (1988). *An Introduction to the Social History of Nursing.* London, Routledge.

Duffield, C., Roche, M., O'Brien-Pallas, L., Aisbett, C., King, M., Aisbett, K. and J. Hall (2007). *Glueing it Together: Nurses, their Work Environment and Patient Safety.* Sydney, University of Technology, Sydney: Centre for Health Services Management.

Emery, F.E. and E.L. Trist (1965). 'The causal texture of organizational environments.' *Human Relations* 18: 21–32.

Evetts, J. (2011). 'A new professionalism? Challenges and opportunities.' *Current Sociology* 59: 406–422.

Finger, S., Gardner, E. and E. Subrahmanian (1993). Design support systems for concurrent engineering: a case study in large power transformer design. International Conference Engineering Design, ICED The Hague.

Flynn, M. and M. McKeown (2009). 'Nurse staffing levels revisited: a consideration of key issues in nurse staffing levels and skill mix research.' *Journal of Nursing Management* 17: 759–766.

Foucault, M. (1973). *The Birth of the Clinic: An Archaeology of Medical Perception.* New York, Vintage Books.

Future Hospital Commission (2013). *Future Hospital: Caring for Medical Patients: A Report from the Future Hospital Commission to the Royal College of Physicians.* London, Royal College of Physicians.

Gamarnikow, E. (1984). 'Nineteenth century nursing reform and the sexual division of labour.' *Bulletin of the History Group of the Royal College of Nursing* 4 **Spring.**
—— (1991). Nurse or woman: gender and professionalism in reformed nursing 1860–1923. *Anthropology and Nursing.* P. Holden and J. Littleworth. London, Routledge: 110–129.

Garrety, K. and R. Badham (2000). 'The politics of socio-technical intervention: an interactionist view.' *Technology Analysis and Strategic Management* 12(1): 103–118.

Gittel, J.H. and L. Weiss (2004). 'Coordination networks within and across organizations: a multi-level framework.' *Journal of Management Studies* 41(1): 127–153.

Goodwin, C. (1995). 'Seeing in depth.' *Social Studies of Science* 25: 237–274.

Ham, C., Dixon, A. and B. Brooke (2012). *Transforming the Delivery of Health and Social Care: The Case for Fundamental Change.* London, The King's Fund.

Heath, C. and N. Staudenmayer (2000). 'Coordination neglect: how lay theories of organizing complicate coordination in organizations.' *Research in Organizational Behaviour* 22: 155–193.

House of Commons (2013). Report of the Mid Staffordshire NHS Foundation Trust Public Inquiry, Volumes I, II and III (Chaired by Robert Francis QC), HC 898. London, The Stationery Office.

Hoyle, E. and P.D. John (1995). *Professional Knowledge and Professional Practice.* London, Cassell.

Imison, C. and R. Bohmer (2013). *NHS and Social Care Workforce: Meeting our Needs Now and in the Future?* London, The King's Fund.

Jacob, E.R., Mckenna, L. and A. D'Amore (2013). 'The changing skill mix in nursing: considerations for and against different levels of nurse.' *Journal of Nursing Management.* Article first published online: 23 Sep 2013: DOI: 10.1111/jonm.12162.

Mackintosh, N. and J. Sandall (2010). 'Short Report: Overcoming gendered and professional hierarchies in order to facilitate escalation of care in emergency situations: the role of standardised communication tools.' *Social Science & Medicine* 71: 1683–1686.

Maitlis, S. and T.B. Lawrence (2007). 'Triggers and enablers of sensegiving in organizations.' *Academy of Management Journal* 50(1): 57–84.

May, C. (1992). 'Nursing work, nurses' knowledge, and the subjectification of the patient.' *Sociology of Health & Illness* 14(4): 472–487.

Melia, K.M. (1979). 'A sociological approach to the analysis of nursing work.' *Journal of Advanced Nursing* 4: 57–67.

Meyer, J.W. and B. Rowan (1977). 'Institutionalized organizations: formal structure as myth and ceremony.' *American Journal of Sociology* 83: 340–363.

Middleton, D. and S.D. Brown (2005). Net-working on a neonatal intensive care unit: the baby as a virtual object. *Actor-Network Theory and Organizing*. B. Czarniawska and T. Hernes. Malmo, Sweden, Liber and Copenhagen Business School Press: 307–328.

Mol, A. (2002). *The Body Multiple: Ontology in Medical Practice*. Durham, NC, Duke University Press.

Munkvold, G. and G. Ellingsen (2007). Common information spaces along the illness trajectories of chronic patients, ECSCW07 Proceedings of the tenth European Conference on Computer Supported Cooperative Work, Limerick, Ireland.

NHS Confederation (2013). *Challenging Bureaucracy*. London, The NHS Confederation.

Nonaka, I. and H. Takeuchi (1995). *The Knowledge-Creating Company*, New York, Oxford University Press, Inc.

Pentland, B.T. and H.H. Reuter (1994). 'Organizational routines as grammars of action.' *Administrative Science Quarterly* 39: 484–510.

Royal College of Nursing (2013). *Paperwork and Administration*. London, Royal College of Nursing.

Simpson, A. (2005). 'Community psychiatric nurses and the care co-ordinator role: squeezed to provide "limited nursing".' *Journal of Advanced Nursing* 52(6): 689–699.

Star, S. and J. Griesemer (1989). 'Institutional ecology, "translations" and boundary objects: amateurs and professionals in Berkely's Museum of Vertebrate Zoology, 1907–39.' *Social Studies of Science* 19: 387–420.

Strauss, A., Schatzman, L., Bucher, R., Ehrlich, D. and M. Sabshin. (1964). *Psychiatric Ideologies and Institutions*. New Brunswick, Transaction Publishers.

Strauss, A., Fagerhaugh, S., Suczet, B and C. Wiener (1985). The Social Organization of Medical Work. Chicago: University of Chicago Press.

Traynor, M. (2009). 'Indeterminacy and technicality revisited: how medicine and nursing have responded to the evidence based movement.' *Sociology of Health & Illness* 31(4): 494–507.

Weick, K.E. (1979). *The Social Psychology of Organizing*. London, Random House.

Index